Introduction

Do you believe your body has the wisdom to heal?

I do. And our symptoms are giving us a heads up to pay attention to our physical, emotional and spiritual needs. Dis-ease is our body telling us there is either emotional congestion to address, physical ailments to nurture and accept versus judge and diminish.

Most of my clients, including myself didn't always speak kindly to my body. Whether it is because of weight, or always falling off the diet, or judging body parts for not being good enough. Now, self-compassion and self-understanding are the two main ingredients to help heal us our mind, body and soul.
Hello, I am Heather Fleming. A Midwest mermaid who is sharing my journey to embrace my feelings of trying to be a perfectionist, a recovering people-pleaser, and my rebellious side when relating to food and this complicated thing called life.

Here are a few of my personal stories to help you tune into trusting your true feelings.

The first day of school was always one of my favorite days of the year. I would get so excited to wear the new clothes that my mom and I purchased in the big city, Sioux City, Iowa. I would get to school, and I could barely sit in my seat from the excitement of seeing my friends, having new experiences, and observing how to behave in this world.

Then a couple of weeks later, the sneeze attacks hit. I had horrible allergies and hay fever. I would bring my extra-large box of Kleenex with lotion so I wouldn't chafe my nose. As I sat at my desk trying to manage my sneezes by either holding them in or catching them in the tissue, the embarrassment and shame would take over. One time I even dislocated my ribs from trying to cover up and hold back sneezing. This inconvenience led me to my first chiropractor visit which I believe 'set' the tone for what would unfold in my future.

I left the Midwest in my late 20's, took my Bachelor's degree in Nutritional Science and began my next chapter in San Diego, California as a Holistic Integrative Nutritionist. One of my lead jokes when I present is, "I had to leave Nebraska because I was allergic to it". (This may or may not be the title of my next book.)

On my 3rd day in San Diego, I met someone who hadn't worked for an entire year. I didn't know this was an option in the game of life. In Husker-land (the sports name for Nebraska), you would have been exiled from the state for being lazy, a detriment to society, and a loser. This person resembled none of these qualities. I began to reflect on my true priorities. This good girl from Nebraska was reassessing what her true values were versus the ones that were passed down from family and society to each generation.

⦿⦿⦿⦿⦿⦿⦿⦿⦿⦿⦿⦿

When did feelings become confusing for you?

Did you know we have over twenty-two senses? Besides the major five and the sixth, there are signals and sensations our body is constantly giving us.

Jill Bolte said it best, "We are FEELING creatures who think", not the other way around. Why did we shut down our feelings and use our minds as our source of discernment? Society? Definition of success? Survival? You are weak if you are sensitive? To be loved and accepted by your family or friends?

As an only child, a bit of a free-spirited Pollyanna and beginning school at a young age, I always felt behind or like I was missing something. This feeling was deep inside me, and I could never put a finger on it until my adult years.

A feeling of shame that ruled my life and choices. This feeling would grip my unconscious and cause me to feel lost, abandoned and alone. These thoughts, feelings and behaviors become our subconscious programming from the ages 0–8. Have you ever seen the movie, "Inside Out"? A little girl moves to another city and has complicated feelings that challenge her core values. We then operate from these values through our adulthood, which can leave us having challenging relationships and feelings of disconnection and confusion.

After many rounds of antibiotics into my teenage years, I went to the dermatologist to tackle the acne. This resulted in two rounds of Acutane, which correlated with taking birth control pills at the same time to avoid pregnancy. The reason for the birth control pills was to prevent a baby from being deformed from the strength of Vitamin A in the medicine. I already had digestive issues before all of this and now all the side effects from these medicines. Almost every time

I ate, I would feel tremendously bloated and had loose stool daily. You can see how this love/dislike relationship with food led me to study what I needed to heal the most: My gut health, my gut intuition, and that underlying repressed emotion that was roaring inside.

Looking back, my repressed feelings, shame and pain were manifesting into physical ailments at a very young age. And to this day, I FULLY believe that our emotional and physical bodies go hand and hand as much as science and metaphysics*.

*(Derived from the Greek meta-ta-physika ("after the things of nature"); referring to an idea, doctrine, or posited reality outside of human sense perception. In modern philosophical terminology, metaphysics refers to the studies of what cannot be reached through objective studies of material reality.

I was aiming to become a raw food, paleo, vegan, holier-than-thou, perfect nutritionist. Well, that caused heaps of anxiety, shame, guilt, and stress, until one day I had my first a-ha.
What if our bodies were brilliant and we trained ourselves on how to listen and understand them? This free-spirited, science-nerd was on her way!

When the book, "Women Who Run with Wolves" came into my life, the roar inside me connected with the yearning for belonging. And the shame pattern became clear.

I belonged to life.

Life was my ultimate love.

Whether you call it God, love, flowers, Universe, Divine, or anything else, this was my ultimate relationship. Now, I had to be brave enough to commit and own the complexity of this beloved relationship.

When I discovered our intuition can be measured by science, my nutrition program became exactly what I wanted to share in the world. Currently, I am studying my love of food by applying Ayurvedic principles, nutritional science regarding the vagus nerve, Polyvagal theory, and nervous system practices to implement into each of my programs. Our nervous system is wired to anticipate our needs by helping our brain and gut connect and relay information to each other.

Most people are trying to outthink their health, while the body is gently nudging us with cues that most do not know how to interpret. Whether we have a gut feeling that prevents us from danger or a hunch which food to choose to provide nourishment and healing to our cells, this is the new program to follow.

Instead of following a restricted or extreme program, you will learn to follow YOU!

The Conscious Nutrition philosophy, simple tips, way of being, thinking, reasoning, and living is for all the rebellious, emotional, sensitive people who feel deeply, liberating the good girl or boy who wants to develop their own personalized program in self-trust.

I do NOT want to expend any more energy trying to live a life that doesn't align with my true values and beliefs. Instead, when we live a nourishing and abundant inner life, then our generosity, compassion and kindness will spread OUT to others.

Thank you for joining me in this independent, self-supporting program to help guide you to TRUST the MOST important person I know, YOU.

Enjoy learning about your Food Relationship Type, Feel Your Meal process, the Conscious Nutrition Food Tree and yummy recipes!

With abundant nourishment,
Heather Fleming, C.C.N.
ConsciousNutrition.com

CONSCIOUS RECIPES

Welcome!

Welcome to the Conscious Nutrition Recipe book. Food is part of our life through health, celebration, community and comfort. These recipes allow you choose high quality foods to support you and your family.

These recipes are in collaboration the Conscious Nutrition Program. I want others to live a life of vitality and joy. When you feed and nourish your body, you will prevent disease symptoms and have more energy to contribute more of yourself in this world.

These are not your typical recipes. These recipes help you connect with your body and organs. Did you know that when you crave certain flavors, textures and temperatures that your organs are giving you hints for what they need to functions?

As you scroll through the recipes, take note of which ones jump out at you, your body needs these ingredients to be more balanced.

Tune into your body and practice the Feel Your Meal process to decide what you are craving? Then, choose a meal that associates with this craving.

Each recipe is broken down by:
1. Flavor Type: Either Sweet or Savory (rich, spicy, or salty)
2. Temperature Type: Either hot or Cold. Do you know the feeling when you want soup versus a salad? This is your body craving homeostasis.
3. Meal Types: Review the Conscious Nutrition Food Tree to choose which Meal Type you prefer. Try rotating these Meal Types and observe your energy, bowel movements, sleep, feelings of guilt, and bloating.

With abundant nourishment,

Heather Fleming

Heather Fleming, C.C.N., Nourishment Leader

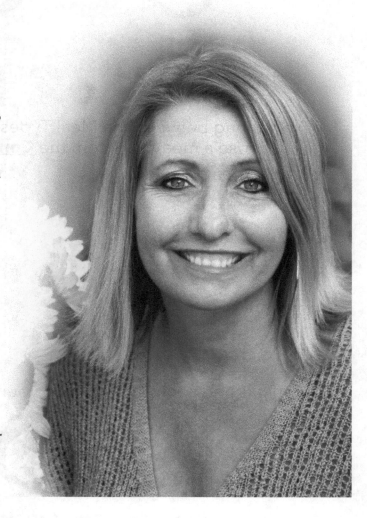

FEEL *Your* MEAL

*Before each meal, meal planning, or grocery shop, practice
these 3-Steps to help you connect to your senses & inner knowing.*

STEP 1 FEEL

HOT or **COLD** and **SWEET** or **SAVORY** (spicy, salty, rich)
Take 5 deep breaths and place your hand on your heart to see if your body
wants a hot or cold meal that contains sweet or savory.

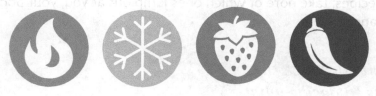

STEP 2 MEAL

Try rotating between the Meal Types at different times of the day.
Choose a meal type from the **Conscious Nutrition Food Tree**

PROTEIN   **STARCH**   **COMBINED**   **VEGAN**

STEP 3 HEAL

After meals and each day, observe your poop, sleep and energy levels.

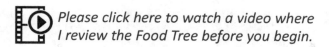 *Please click here to watch a video where I review the Food Tree before you begin.*

CONSCIOUS NUTRITION
FOOD TREE

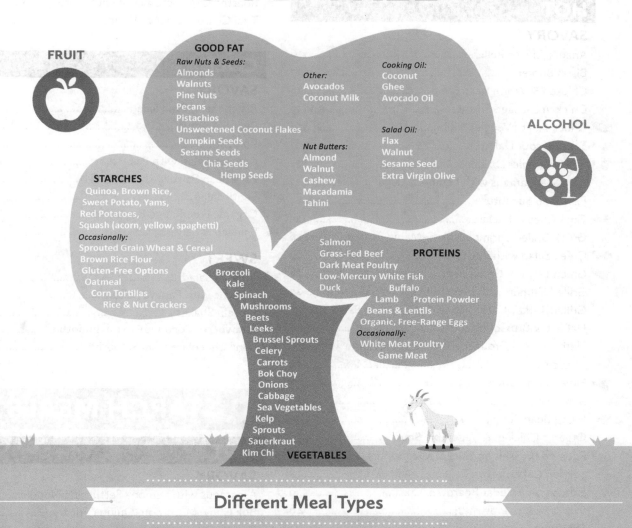

FRUIT

GOOD FAT

Raw Nuts & Seeds:
Almonds
Walnuts
Pine Nuts
Pecans
Pistachios
Unsweetened Coconut Flakes
Pumpkin Seeds
Sesame Seeds
Chia Seeds
Hemp Seeds

Other:
Avocados
Coconut Milk

Nut Butters:
Almond
Walnut
Cashew
Macadamia
Tahini

Cooking Oil:
Coconut
Ghee
Avocado Oil

Salad Oil:
Flax
Walnut
Sesame Seed
Extra Virgin Olive

ALCOHOL

STARCHES
Quinoa, Brown Rice,
Sweet Potato, Yams,
Red Potatoes,
Squash (acorn, yellow, spaghetti)
Occasionally:
Sprouted Grain Wheat & Cereal
Brown Rice Flour
Gluten-Free Options
Oatmeal
Corn Tortillas
Rice & Nut Crackers

PROTEINS
Salmon
Grass-Fed Beef
Dark Meat Poultry
Low-Mercury White Fish
Duck
Buffalo
Lamb   Protein Powder
Beans & Lentils
Organic, Free-Range Eggs
Occasionally:
White Meat Poultry
Game Meat

Broccoli
Kale
Spinach
Mushrooms
Beets
Leeks
Brussel Sprouts
Celery
Carrots
Bok Choy
Onions
Cabbage
Sea Vegetables
Kelp
Sprouts
Sauerkraut
Kim Chi
VEGETABLES

Different Meal Types

Try rotating between Protein, Starch, Vegan and Combined Meals. Try different meal combinations at different times of the day to see what best supports your body and energy.

 Protein Meals are the right side of the Conscious Nutrition Food Tree combined with healthy fat and vegetables.

 Combined Meals are protein combined with a starch in the same meal complemented with veggies and fat.

 Starch Meals are on the left side of the Conscious Nutrition Food Tree combined with healthy fat and vegetables.

 Vegan Meals
Veggies combined with fats or Fruit combined with a fat.

Contents

PROTEIN MEALS

HOT

SAVORY

SWEET

HOT Continued

SWEET

COLD

SAVORY

SWEET

STARCH MEALS

HOT

SAVORY

Contents

Contents

VEGAN MEALS
CONTINUED

SNACKS

DRESSINGS

DESSERTS

DRINKS

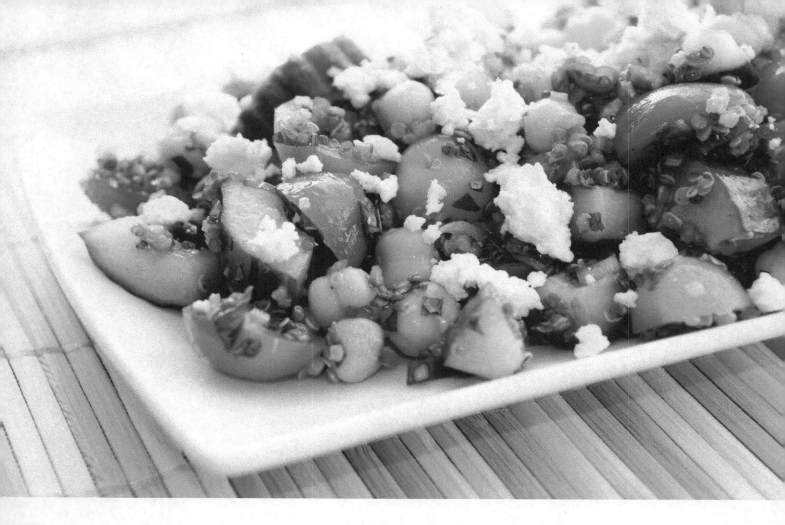

🐾 Protein Meal Recipes

There are many popular high protein diets. Protein is essential for health. However, meat can be difficult to digest in large quantities for some people who have a compromised digestive system.

Proteins need healthy stomach acid to break down properly. If you have digestive issues after protein meals, you may need more support. The goal of separating proteins from starch may help your body feel better after meals.

There are many protein meals available with a variety of vegetarian options.

Enjoy!

Anahi's Chilles Rellenos

(60 Minutes)

A dear friend's and the designer of my logo's recipe.

🔥 SERVED HOT

🌙 SAVORY

INGREDIENTS:

Chiles Poblanos (Wide & Flat)	**4**
Red Onion	**1/2** (finely chopped)
Zucchinis	**2** (finely shredded)
Rotisserie Chicken Shredded	**1** thigh / **1** breast

FOR THE GREEN SAUCE:

Tomatillos (small green Mexican tomatoes that come with a dry skin that needs to be peeled)	**10**
Chicken Or Vegetable Broth	**½** cup
Garlic	**3** cloves
Yellow Onion	**½** small onion
Dry Cilantro	**1** tbs
Jalapeno Pepper	**1**
Sea Salt & Pepper (To Taste)	

1 Start by charting the Chiles Poblanos in the stove. Make sure you turn around the chiles with some tongs so the skin gets burn evenly. After all chiles are well charted, place the chiles in a plastic bag so they sweat and let them rest in the back for about 20 to 30 minutes.

2 Then open the bag and under warm water peel off all the burnt skin of the chiles, the chiles are very delicate so it has to be done very carefully. Open each chile with a knife with a small long cut and carefully remove the seeds and veins so they don't blow your head off from spice. On a wok, cook the onion with a table spoon of olive oil and add the shredded zucchini, season with sea salt and pepper. Mix in the shredded chicken and set aside.

3 Carefully, fill in the chiles with the chicken mix and close chiles with a wood toothpick. Assemble all chiles and set them aside.

4 Prepare a deep pot with a steamer rack and place the chiles to steam for about 10 minutes once the water is boiling.

Sauce

1 Chart all the tomatillos and cut them into small pieces. On a sauce pan, sauté onions and garlic and add the tomatillos after charted. Then add the broth and jalapeño pepper.

2 Sea salt and pepper to taste and the dry cilantro. Let the sauce cook and reduce a bit for about 20 minutes in a gentle boil. After the chiles are steamed, place them on a platter and cover them with the green sauce and they are ready to eat!

3 You can sprinkle some fresh Cotija Mexican cheese which is super light and only sprinkle it as a garnish. I don't put any cheese to make them dairy free but they are nice with it too.

Buen Provecho!

Bison Burger

(15 Minutes)

INGREDIENTS:

Ground Bison (Buffalo)	2 lbs
Finely Chopped Fresh Sage	2 tbl
Sea Salt	1½ tspn
Black Pepper	2 tspn
Onion (Finely Chopped)	½
Olive Oil	2 tbl

Buffalo is a great alternative for beef with more iron, vitamin B, Omega 3's and less saturated fat.

🔥 SERVED HOT

🌙 SAVORY

1 Sauté the onions in the olive oil over low-medium heat until translucent. Turn off the heat and let it cool.

2 When the onions are cool enough to touch, gently mix them in with the bison burger meat, and add everything else. Do not overwork the meat, it will result in a tough burger. Just gently fold it until the onions, sage, sea salt and pepper are well mixed in.

3 Form patties with the meat, using about 1/4 to 1/3 of a pound of meat per patty. Here's a tip on making the patty: if you press a slight indentation in the center of each patty it will help keep the burgers in a nice disk shape when cooking. Otherwise the burger will start to get a little egg-shaped as the edges contract from cooking.

4 Grill or fry the burgers on medium heat, about 6-7 minutes per side, less or more depending on the thickness of the burger and the heat of the pan/grill, or until the internal temperature is 140° F for medium rare, or 160° F for well done.

Chicken & White Bean Soup

(15 Minutes)

This soup is hearty and has extra protein with the chicken and bean combination. Make a big pot over the weekend to have ready during the busier time of the week.

🔥 SERVED HOT

🌙 SAVORY

INGREDIENTS:

Olive Oil	**2** tspn
Leeks White And Light Green Parts Only, Cut Into 1/4-Inch Rounds	**2**
Chopped Fresh Sage or ¼ Teaspoon Dried	**1** tbl
Reduced-Sodium Chicken Broth 2 (14-Ounce) Cans	
Water	**2** cups
Cannellini Beans, Rinsed (15-Ounce) Can	**1**
Roasted Chicken Skin Discarded, Meat Removed From Bones And Shredded	**4** cups

1 Heat oil in a Dutch oven over medium-high heat. Add leeks and cook, stirring often, until soft, about 3 minutes. Stir in sage and continue cooking until aromatic, about 30 seconds. Stir in broth and water, increase heat to high, cover and bring to a boil. Add beans, chicken, and cook, uncovered, stirring occasionally, until heated through, about 3 minutes. Serve hot.

Chicken Sausage Frittata

(55 Minutes)

INGREDIENTS:

Olive Oil	**2** tbl
Yellow Onion (Peeled & Sliced)	**1** small
Chicken Sausage	**3–4** links
Spinach	**1** cup
Organic Free Range Eggs	**3**
Sea Salt & Freshly Ground Black Pepper	
Fresh Thyme Leaves (Optional)	**1** lg pinch

This is one of my favorite meals to make and re-heat through out the week for a quick breakfast.

◑ SERVED HOT

◑ SAVORY

1   Preheat the oven to 350° F. Layer in a glass pan, the onions, spinach and sausages, seasoning with sea salt and pepper as you go. Add beaten organic free range eggs. Bake in the oven until the eggs are set, about 45 minutes.

Chock Full of Veggies Chili

(45 Minutes)

If you have the chili craving and do not want the meat.

🔥 SERVED HOT

🌑 SAVORY

INGREDIENTS:

Extra Virgin Olive Oil	1 tbl
Red Bell Peppers Chopped	2
Chopped Mushrooms	1½ cups
Onion, Chopped	1 large
Celery, Chopped	2 stalks
Garlic, Minced	3 cloves
Chili Powder	1 tbl
Dried Oregano	1 tbl
Ground Cumin	1 tspn
Sea Salt	¼ tspn
Pinto Beans	2 15 oz cans
No-Salt Added Diced Tomatoes, With Juices	14½ oz can

1 In a large saucepan, heat oil over medium heat. Add peppers, mushrooms, onion, celery and garlic; cook, stirring until vegetables begin to soften, about 7 minutes. Add chili powder, oregano, cumin, and sea salt; cook, stirring occasionally, 5 minutes more.

2 Add beans and tomatoes with their juices. Bring to a gentle simmer and cook, stirring occasionally, until chili is fragrant and slightly thickened, 25 to 30 minutes. Serve warm.

Easy Masoor Dal

(40 Minutes if you soak lentils first for 2 hours)

INGREDIENTS:

Red Lentils	**1**	cup
Ginger (1 Inch Piece, Peeled)	**1**	slice
Ground Turmeric	**¼**	tspn
Sea Salt	**1**	tspn
Cayenne Pepper (Or To Taste)	**½**	tspn
Olive Oil	**4**	tspn
Dried Minced Onion	**4**	tspn
Cumin Seeds	**1**	tspn

Dal is a low inflammatory protein meal, and great for vegetarians. If you add rice, it is a combined meal.

◉ SERVED HOT

◉ SAVORY

1 Rinse lentils thoroughly and place in a medium saucepan along with ginger, turmeric, sea salt and cayenne pepper. Cover with about 1 inch of water and bring to a boil. Skim off any foam that forms on top of the lentils. Reduce heat and simmer, stirring occasionally, until beans are tender and soupy.

2 Combine oil, dried onion and cumin seeds until brown in another pan. Stir into lentil mixture.

Egg Scrambles

(20 Minutes)

⬥ SERVED HOT   🍓 SWEET   ⬥ SERVED HOT   🍃 SAVORY

Scrambles are easy to prepare for a conscious breakfast and to start your day with vegetables.

This meal can be as quick as grab and go, and definitely more supportive to start your day off right.

Conscious Egg Scramble

Egg White Scramble

INGREDIENTS:

Organic Free Range	1 egg
Organic Free Range Egg Whites	½ cup
Zucchini Diced	½
Mushrooms	½ cup
Spinach	1 cup
Coconut Oil	½ tbl
Avocado	½

Add Other Vegetables You Desire, Try To Incorporate 2 Cups Total (Be Cautious Of Night Shade Vegetables)

1. Add 1/2 tablespoon of coconut oil to warm pan. Add vegetables and slightly sauté. Add organic free range egg and organic free range egg white mixture.
2. Cook lightly, top with avocado, add sea salt and pepper to taste.

INGREDIENTS:

Organic Free Range Egg Whites	1 cup
Chopped Veggies Of Your Choice	
Coconut Oil	1 tspn
Sea Salt & Pepper (To Taste)	

1. Heat oil in pan and sauté vegetables. Add organic free range egg whites, scramble and season.

Filet & Asparagus with Lemon & Organic Ghee

(17 Minutes)

INGREDIENTS:

Medium Filet Steaks	**2**
Garlic, Chopped	**2** cloves
Asparagus	**10** Spears
Worcestershire Sauce	**¼** cup
Mustard	**¼** cup
Olive Oil	**¼** cup
Ghee (Clarified Butter)	
Lemon Juice	**1** tbl
Sea Salt & Pepper (To Taste)	

When you crave a steak, your body may need it. Try to purchase grass-fed beef from a conscious resource you trust.

🔥 SERVED HOT

🌿 SAVORY

1 Make a marinade by combining Worcestershire sauce, olive oil, and mustard together in a bowl. Cover flank steaks in marinade, and set in fridge for 15 minutes.

2 While flank steaks are marinating, cut white ends off of asparagus. Cook asparagus in ghee (Clarified Butter) and squeeze lemon juice over medium heat for 10 minutes, rotating every couple minutes to not burn sides.

3 After marinating flank steaks, cook steaks in skillet over medium-high heat in olive oil for 3 minutes on each side

4 Plate steaks and asparagus, season with salt and pepper, and serve!

Fish Taco Substitute

(15 Minutes)

We love fish tacos in San Diego. Here is a protein meal option to support less feelings of bloating and food coma.

🔥 SERVED HOT

🌑 SAVORY

Mahi-Mahi
(4 Ounce Portion Per Person)

Lemon	**1** whole
Refried Beans	**1** cup
Shredded Cabbage	**1** cup
Salsa Fresca (See Recipe On Page 14)	**½** cup
Avocado	**1** whole

1   Marinate Mahi-mahi in lemon and season. Sauté for 4-5 minutes on each side. Top with shredded cabbage, avocado, and salsa fresca. Add re-fried beans on the side.

Goat Cheese Frittata

(30 Minutes)

MEAL TYPE:

Protein Meal

INGREDIENTS:

Finely Chopped Onion	⅓ cup
Thinly Sliced Zucchini	1 cup
Finely Chopped Red Bell Pepper	½ cup
Finely Chopped Orange Bell Pepper	½ cup
Olive Oil	1½ tbl
Organic Eggs	4 large
Minced Fresh Parsley Leaves	2 tbl

*A satiating
protein breakfast, perfect for a
weekend brunch.*

🔥 SERVED HOT

🧅 SAVORY

1 In a 9-inch non-stick skillet cheat 1 T oil olive oil, cook the onion, the zucchini, and the peppers with salt and black pepper to taste for 10 minutes until vegetables are soft.

2 In a bowl whisk together the eggs and the parsley,, add the vegetable mixture, and stir the mixture until it is combined well.

3 In the skillet heat the remaining 1/2 tablespoon oil over moderate heat until it is hot but not smoking, pour in the egg mixture, distributing the vegetables evenly, and cook the frittata, without stirring, for 8 to 10 minutes, or until the edge is set but the center is still soft.

Greek Grilled Shrimp or Mahi-Mahi

(30 Minutes)

This is a great light meal to support quality protein intake.

🔥 SERVED HOT

🌿 SAVORY

INGREDIENTS:

Shrimp Or Mahi-Mahi	1 lb
Olive Oil	1½ cup
Lemons, Juiced	2
Garlic, Minced	3 cloves
Fresh Thyme, Chopped	1 tbl
Fresh Rosemary, Chopped	1 tbl
Fresh Oregano, Chopped	1 tbl
Lemon Pepper Seasoning	½ tspn

1 Combine fresh herbs, olive oil, garlic, lemon pepper, and lemon juice in a large container. Add shrimp (or Mahi-mahi) to mixture, cover container, and allow marinating overnight in refrigerator.

2 Preheat grill for high heat. Remove shrimp (or Mahi-mahi) from marinade and place on lightly oiled grate. Cook 5-7 minutes per side. Remove from grill and serve immediately.

Greek Salad with Zucchini

(30 Minutes)

INGREDIENTS:

Zucchini, Cut In ½ & Then Cut In 1 Inch Thick Slices	**3** medium
Grape Tomatoes Or Roma Tomatoes Cut In Quarters	**4** cups
Organic Dried Dill	**1** tbl
Organic Olive Oil	**3** tbl
Balsamic Vinegar	**2** tbl
Romaine Lettuce Torn Into Bite-Size Pieces	**2** bunches
Crumbled Feta Cheese	**4** oz
Kalamata Olives, Pitted	**¼** cup
Sea Salt & Pepper (To Taste)	

Feta has a bit of protein in it, and dairy combines best with proteins, vegetables and fat vs. starch and fruit.

🔥 SERVED HOT

⚫ SAVORY

1   Heat broiler. In a medium bowl, add zucchini, tomatoes, dill, 1 tablespoon of organic olive oil and sea salt and pepper. Toss together to coat. Place on cookie sheet and broil until slightly charred, 15 -25 minutes. Remove when edges are browned and transfer to a plate to cool. Wipe cookie sheet clean with a paper towel and set aside.

2   In a glass bowl, combine vinegar, remaining olive oil, sea salt and pepper to taste. Whisk together until combined.

3   Place lettuce, zucchini mixture, feta cheese and olive in bowl and toss with salad dressing. Serve at once.

Green Lentil & Green Bean Casserole

(60 Minutes)

I am in love with this casserole. A client gave me the idea and now it keeps getting better every time I make it
Craving Type: This dish can help with umami cravings
(craving something meaty)

🔥 SERVED HOT

⚫ SAVORY

MEAL TYPE:

Vegetarian/Dairy Protein Meal

INGREDIENTS:

Green Lentils	**1** cup
Vegetable Broth	**3** cups
Bay Leaf	**1** leaf
Carrot, Chopped	**1** large
Celery, Chopped	**2** ribs
Onion, Chopped	**1** small
Yellow Or Red Bell Pepper	**1** small
Zucchini	**1** small
Garlic, Minced	**1** clove
Salt	**½** tspn
Ground Black Pepper	**¼** tspn
Goat Cheese	**6** oz

1 Before cooking the lentils, make sure you rinse them well and pick over them to remove any small rocks or debris. Combine lentils, chicken broth and bay leaf in a medium saucepan. Bring to a boil, then turn heat down and simmer until lentils are tender, 25-30 minutes for French green lentils or 20-25 minutes for common brown or green lentils.

2 Sauté onion and garlic then add the remainder of the vegetables and cook for 5 minutes. Add vegetables into a casserole dish, top with cooked lentils. Stir and chunk up the goat cheese into the mixture. Bake for 20 minutes. Serve!

Grilled Salmon with Herbed Lentils & Salsa Verde

(50 Minutes)

Another meal with extra high quality protein foods combined to enhance flavor and nutrition.

⬤ SERVED HOT   ⬤ SAVORY

FOR THE HERB LENTILS:

Lentils	**7** oz
Fresh Sage Leaves	**4**
Fresh Flat-Leaf Parsley	**3** Stems
Celery	**1** rib
Olive Oil	**4** tbl
Red Wine Vinegar	**1** tbl
Fresh Dill, Chopped	**2** sprigs
Fresh Flat-Leaf Parsley, Chopped	**3** sprigs
Fresh Basil, Chopped	**3** sprigs
Sea Salt & Freshly Ground Black Pepper	
Grated Zest & Juice Of **1** Lemon	

FOR THE SALSA VERDE:

Garlic	**1** clove
Capers, Rinsed	**2** tbl
Dijon Mustard	**1** tspn
Fresh Basil	**3** sprigs
Fresh Mint	**3** Sprigs
Leaves From Fresh Flat-Leaf Parsley (Stems Reserved For The Herb Lentils)	**3** Sprigs
Red Wine Vinegar	**1** tbl
Olive Oil	**3** tbl
Juice Of **1/2** Lemon	
Olive Oil, For Grilling	
Salmon Fillets, 1 Portion-Sized Piece Per Person, Skin On	

1 First make the herb lentils. In a pan, cover the lentils with cold water and bring to a summer over medium heat. Add the sage leaves, parsley stems, and celery. Simmer until the lentils are al dente, and then remove from the heat and drain, reserving a little of the cooking water. Discard the celery and herbs.

2 Season the lentils while hot with sea salt and black pepper, and add the oil, vinegar, and the lemon juice and zest, so they will better absorb all the flavors. When the lentils have cooled, add the chopped herbs.

3 For the salsa Verde, place the garlic and capers in Emulsifying Blender until smooth. Add the Dijon mustard and all the herbs, then purée until you have a smooth green paste. Add the lemon juice and red wine vinegar, and then stir in the olive oil. Check the seasoning and add more sea salt, pepper, and lemon juice, if necessary.

4 Place a lightly oiled, heavy-bottomed griddle pan over medium to high heat. Season the salmon fillets with sea salt and black pepper and place in the pan, skin-side down. Grill the salmon for 4 minutes until crisp. Roll the fish over and cook for 2 minutes on each of the other sides. When cooking salmon you want the flesh to be medium-rare in the center; the residual heat will continue cooking the fish after it has been removed from the heat.

Serve the grilled fish with the herb lentils and the salsa Verde, perhaps alongside some other vegetables or a mixed peppery leaf salad.

Grilled Turkey Carpaccio with Asparagus Salad

(40 Minutes)

*Another great turkey meal besides just Thanksgiving.
Turkey can provide essential amino acids and supports our neurotransmitters*

🔥 SERVED HOT

🌙 SAVORY

INGREDIENTS:

Turkey Breasts Pounded Thin Into Round Flat Cutlets (Ask Your Butcher To Slice The Boneless Turkey Breast Thin)	**4** 6 oz
Leek	**1**
Garlic	**2** cloves
Sun Chokes Peeled & Rough Chopped	**1** cup
Homemade Chicken Stock	**1** cup
White Wine	**¼** cup
Chopped Fresh Thyme	**2** tbl
Dijon Mustard	**1** tspn
Capers Rinsed	**1** tspn
Pomegranate Molasses	**2** tspn
Olive Oil	**½** cup
Large Asparagus	**1** bunch
Meyer Lemon Juice	**¼** cup
Fresh Lemon Zest	**½** tspn
Frisee	**½** Head

1 Season the cutlets with the half of the lemon zest and a pinch of the thyme with sea salt and pepper. In a medium saucepot, sauté sun chokes 1 tbsp thyme, garlic, and leek, for about 4-5 minutes deglaze with white wine reduce for about 1-2 minutes add stock season well. Simmer until sun chokes are tender. In Emulsifying Blender, strain the sun choke mixture then puree, season if needed.

2 Add back to a pot and keep warm. In a bowl, add the remaining thyme, Dijon mustard, pomegranate molasses, and the lemon juice. Season with sea salt and pepper and slowly drizzle in olive oil, add capers and adjust seasoning. Shave asparagus thin with a knife or a peeler in long strips toss with the frisee and a few tspn of the vinaigrette and season with sea salt and pepper. Grill the turkey cutlets about 2-3 minutes per side depending upon thickness. Plate with a spoonful of the sun choke puree top with the cutlet, then with the asparagus salad and spoon the vinaigrette around.

Halibut & Brussels Sprouts

(30 Minutes)

INGREDIENTS:

Brussels Sprouts, Outer Leaves Removed And Cut In Half	8-10
Halibut, Skin Removed (6 ounce) portions	2
Olive Oil	
Sea Salt & Pepper (To Taste)	

This is a great brain enhancing meal to have the night before a big meeting or a wanting to feel even sassier in your swimsuit.

◐ SERVED HOT

◐ SAVORY

1. Preheat oven to 375° F, toss halved brussels sprouts with 2 tablespoons olive oil, and season with sea salt and pepper. Place in roasting dish and put in oven for 15 minutes or until outer leaves are crisp and slightly brown and insides are tender. Keep warm.

2. Heat a nonstick skillet over medium high heat and add about 1-2 tablespoons of olive oil to pan. Season both fillets of fish with sea salt and pepper, and add to pan. Sear fish until a light brown crust begins to form, about 5 minutes; flip fish and cook on other side until cooked through, about 4 more minutes.

Herb Crusted Grouper with
Yellow Heirloom Tomato Sauce

(15 Minutes)

🔥 SERVED HOT   🍓 SWEET

This is a simple preparation of fish that relies on the robust flavors of the ingredients. Make sure that your fish is very fresh and of high quality.

FISH INGREDIENTS:

Grouper Filets (⅓ Pound Each)	4
Lemon, Zested	1
Thyme Leaves	1 tbl
Chopped Flat Leaf Parsley	3 tbl
Good Extra Virgin Olive Oil	2 tbl
Kosher Salt (To Taste)	

SAUCE INGREDIENTS:

Ripe Yellow Heirloom Tomatoes	2 lbs
Diced Onion	1 cup
Extra-Virgin Olive Oil	3 tbl
Chopped Basil	¼ cup
Kosher Salt & Fresh Ground Pepper (To Taste)	

FISH DIRECTIONS

1 Rub the fillets with the oil, pat with herbs, lemon zest, and kosher salt. Heat your skillet for a couple minutes, add olive oil, and heat on high. Sauté fish for about 2-3 minutes per side on medium-high heat until cooked through. (The fish should flake easily in the center.) Don't flip the fish more than once. Remove and serve topped with sauce.

SAUCE DIRECTIONS

1 Cut the tomatoes into quarters and add to Emulsifying Blender. Heat skillet, add olive oil, and heat another minute. Add onions, sauté over medium heat until translucent. Add tomatoes and pinch of kosher salt. Sauté 8 minutes over medium heat. Remove from heat; add chopped basil, kosher salt and pepper to taste. Top herb crusted fish with tomato sauce. Serve with roasted potatoes and sautéed collard greens.

Hibernation Bowl

(15 Minutes if you soak beans or 40 if you need to cook them)

INGREDIENTS:

Pinto Beans, Canned Or Dried (Soak For 12 Hours)	1 cup
Brussels Sprouts, Sliced	1 cup
Zucchini, Cubed	½ cup
Spinach	1 cup
Coconut Oil	1 tbl

CHIMICHURRI SAUCE:

1 1/2 Cup Parsley	1½ cup
Lemon	½ lemon
Olive Oil	1 tbl
Red Wine Vinegar	⅓ cup
Garlic	2 cloves

Bowls are a great way to reheat your leftovers and pack them with nutrient-dense foods.

🔥 SERVED HOT

🌶 SAVORY

1   Cook beans in a sauce pan, if canned for a few minutes or if you soaked them, cook for 30 minutes then set aside.

2   Sauté coconut oil and add Brussels sprouts and zucchini until tender. Add in spinach last to wilt.

3   In a large bowl, place the beans and veggies and then top with sauce.

4   Blend the Chimichurri sauce ingredients and enjoy!

Meatloaf

(60 Minutes)

A good ole fashioned meal. I personally crave the texture of meatloaf often. This heart-y meal may help you feel comforted.

⬤ SERVED HOT

⬤ SAVORY

INGREDIENTS:

Olive Oil	1 tbl
Yellow Onions, Chopped (About 3 Cups)	2 medium
Garlic, Minced	3 cloves
Sea Salt	2 tspn
Black Pepper	1 tspn
Chicken Broth	⅓ cup
1 tbl Of Tomato Paste	
Ground Bison (I Recommend A Combination Of 85-96% Lean)	2½ lbs
Of Almond Flour	½ cup
Organic Free Range Eggs, Beaten	2 x-large
Can Of Tomato Sauce	1 (8 oz)

1. Preheat your oven to 325° F. Heat the olive oil in a medium sauté pan. Add the onions and minced garlic and cook over medium-low heat, stirring occasionally, for 8 to 10 minutes, until the onions are translucent but not brown. Turn off the heat, add chicken stock, and tomato paste and allow to cool slightly. In a large bowl, combine the bison, onion mixture, almond flour, sea salt, pepper and organic free range eggs, and mix lightly with a fork. Line a cookie sheet with parchment paper and spread the tomato sauce evenly on top. Bake for 1 to 1 hour and 20 minutes, until the internal temperature is 160° F and the meatloaf is cooked through.

Mung Bean Soup

(50 Minutes)

INGREDIENTS:

Mung Beans Whole Green Or Split Green Or Yellow But Green Is Best	400 g
Water	2 litres
Turmeric Powder	½ tspn
Lime Juice	
Fresh Root Ginger	⅔ tspn
Garlic	2-3 cloves
Half An Onion & Any **Other Vegetables**	
Olive Oil	
Cumin Seeds & **Coriander Seeds** **& Other Spices (To Taste)**	1 tspn ea
Sea Salt (To Taste)	

This soup is very cleansing for your liver and kidneys. It will help remove heat, mucus, and inflammation from your organs.

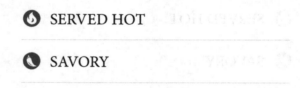 **SERVED HOT**

SAVORY

1 Wash the mung beans thoroughly and then soak them either over night or for at least four hours before cooking. Heat olive oil in a pan and add a teaspoon of turmeric powder. Sauté for a few seconds and then add the soaked beans, fresh water and some fresh root ginger.

2 For one part soaked Mung you need about four parts of water. Leave to bubble away for 30-40 minutes and add more water if necessary. Continue to cook until all the beans are soft and broken up. If you use a pressure cooker, the soup needs cooking for only 8 minutes once the vessel has come to pressure. You can then turn off the heat and leave the pot to cool for a further 10 minutes before opening it.

3 Once the beans are cooked, heat some ghee or olive oil in another pan, add 2-3 cloves of chopped garlic and half a chopped onion and sauté lightly for a minute until soft but still aromatic. Now add some finally chopped fresh root ginger.

4 Next add one teaspoon of cumin and coriander seeds plus any other herbs or spices such as cardamom seeds, black pepper, black cumin seeds etc. and briefly sauté. Add these sautéed spices plus some rock salt into the Mung beans and continue to simmer for a further few minutes. Serve the soup warm with a good squeeze of lime juice, and some fresh coriander leaves, finely chopped and stirred into the soup. If you feel like a little variety, you can also add green leafy vegetables and pumpkin. You can also blend the soup for a better consistency and flavor.

Organic Chicken & Vegetable Soup

(45 Minutes)

*One of my favorite soups when
you feel a bit under the weather.
Your immune system will
be restored to health after a
bowl of this.*

 SERVED HOT

 SAVORY

INGREDIENTS:

Organic Free-Range Chicken (Or Equivalent Weight Of Desired Parts)	**1** whole
Yellow Onion, Chopped	**1** large
Celery With Leaves, Chopped	**2** stalks
Carrot, Peeled & Chopped	**1**
Celery Root, Peeled & Cubed	**1** medium
Parsnip, Peeled & Chopped	**1**
Zucchini, Chopped	**1**
Parsley, Chopped	**½** cup
Bay Leaf	**1** leaf
Black Or White Peppercorns	**5** whole
Sea Salt (To Taste)	

1 Boil 1-1/2 quarts of water in a large soup pot. Thoroughly rinse chicken in cold water and place in pot. Return water to a boil and then reduce heat. Simmer for 10-15 min. until all foam rises to top. Skim foam.

2 Combine all chopped vegetables in a bowl. Once chicken is done simmering and foam removed, carefully add vegetables to the pot. Add bay leaf, peppercorns, and sea salt. Increase heat until simmering again and then lower to maintain low simmer. For maximum flavor, do not boil on high.

3 Simmer for 30-40 minutes, until vegetables are soft. Remove from heat and add chopped parsley. Remove chicken from pot with large utensils and place in a bowl. When cool enough to touch, divide chicken into desired parts or remove all meat and discard skin and bones. Return meat to pot.

4 Serve and enjoy!

Roasted Brussels Sprouts & Mushrooms

(50 Minutes)

*A quick Vegan Meal
to fill up your belly
and your spirit.*

🔥 SERVED HOT

🌙 SAVORY

INGREDIENTS:

Brussels Sprouts, Trimmed & Halved Lengthwise	**3** lb
Olive Oil	¼ cup
Maple Syrup, Grade B	½ cup
Minced Garlic	½ tbl
Sea Salt	
Cracked Pepper	
Olive Oil	**1** cup
Large Shallots (About 6),	½ lb
Cut Crosswise Into 1/8 Inch Thick Slices Separated Intro Rings (2 ½ Cups)	

FOR MUSHROOMS:

Unsalted Butter Or Coconut Oil	¾ stick (6 tbl)
Shiitake Mushrooms Or Mixed Fresh Wild Mushrooms Such As Chanterelle & Oyster, Trimmed, Quartered If Large	1¼ lb
Dry White Wine	¼ cup
Chopped Fresh Thyme	1 tbl
Chopped Fresh Marjoram	1 tbl
Salt	½ tspn
Black Pepper	¼ tspn
Water	½ cup

1 Put oven rack in upper third of oven and preheat oven to 450 F.
2 Line 2 shallow baking sheet with tin foil, and place in oven.
3 Toss Brussels sprouts with olive oil, maple syrup, garlic salt, and pepper.
4 Roast, stirring occasionally and switching position of pans halfway through roasting, until tender, browned, and a little crispy about, 25 to 35 minutes.

Fry Shallots while Brussels Sprouts Roast:

5 Heat oil in a 10-inch heavy skillet over moderate heat until temperature reaches then fry shallots in 3 batches, until golden brown, 3 to 5 minutes per batch
6 Quickly transfer with a slotted spoon to paper towels to drain, spreading in a single layer. Pour off oil from skillet.

Sauté Mushrooms and Assemble Dish:

1 Heat 5 tablespoons butter in skillet over moderately high heat until foam subsides, then sauté mushrooms, stirring occasionally, until golden brown and tender, about 7 minutes.
2 Add wine, thyme, marjoram, salt, and pepper and simmer, uncovered, stirring occasionally, until liquid is reduced to a glaze, about 2 minutes.
3 Add water (1/2 cup) and remaining tablespoon butter and simmer, swirling skillet, until butter is melted.
4 Transfer to a serving dish and stir in Brussels sprouts. Sprinkle with some of shallots and serve with remaining shallots on the side.

Salmon Cakes

(75 Minutes, then chill the cakes)

These are great to have premade to just cook up for a quick and satisfying meal.

🔥 SERVED HOT

🌙 SAVORY

INGREDIENTS:

Fresh Or Frozen Salmon	1-2 lbs
Sweet Onion	½ large
Almond Meal	¼ cup
Organic Free Range Egg	1
Coconut Oil	
Artichoke Hearts	1 can
Roma Tomatoes	2
Sea Salt & Pepper (To Taste)	

1 Blend salmon in Emulsifying Blender and transfer to a mixing bowl

2 Add in artichoke hearts, sweet onion and tomatoes and mix

3 Slowly add in almond meal until you reach the right consistency

4 Dip in organic free range egg.

5 Place in refrigerator for one hour.

6 Heat oil in pan and cook on medium to medium-high heat.

Salmon on a Cedar Board

(30 Minutes after you prep the cedar board)

INGREDIENTS:

Salmon Fillets	**2** lbs
3/4 Thick Cedar Board Big Enough To Hold Fillets	

SEASONING

Fresh Basil	**¼** cup
Fresh Thyme	**1** tspn
Sea Salt & Pepper (To Taste)	

This recipe is great to help you ease-in to any of my programs.

🔥 SERVED HOT

🌿 SAVORY

1   Submerge the cedar board in water the night before. Combine marinade ingredients with salmon and refrigerate for 24 hours.

2   Set barbeque to medium and place cedar onto grill. Place fillets on board flesh side down. Close cover and cook 25 minutes (Salmon should be opaque all the way through).

Salt & Pepper Prawns

(18 Minutes)

Wonderful combination of flavors, you may even feel like you are on vacation.

🔥 SERVED HOT

🌙 SAVORY

INGREDIENTS:

Lime Juice		¼ cup
Braggs Liquid Amino Acids		4 tspn
Sesame Oil		4 tspn
Raw Sugar		1 tspn
Cabbage Preferably Napa, Thinly Sliced (About 1/2 Head)		6 cups
Red Or Orange Bell Peppers, Very Thinly Sliced		2 small
Rice Flour		¼ cup
Kosher Sea Salt		½ tspn
Freshly Ground Pepper		1 tspn
Five-Spice Powder, Chinese Flavoring		1 tspn
Raw Shrimp (21-25 Per Pound), Peeled And Deveined		1⅓ lbs
Olive Oil		2 tbl
Jalapeno Peppers, Seeded & Minced		2

1 Whisk lime juice, soy sauce, sesame oil and sugar in a large bowl until the sugar is dissolved. Add cabbage and bell peppers; toss to combine.

2 Combine rice flour, sea salt, pepper and five-spice powder in a medium bowl. Add shrimp and toss to coat in spice mixture. Heat oil in a large nonstick skillet over medium-high heat. Add the shrimp and cook, stirring often, until pink and curled, 3 to 4 minutes. Add jalapeños and cook until the shrimp are cooked through, about 1 minute more. Serve the slaw topped with the shrimp.

Shakshuka

(30 Minutes)

INGREDIENTS:

Onion, Diced	1 med
Red Bell Pepper, Seeded & Diced	1
Garlic Cloves, Finely Chopped	4 cloves
Paprika	2 tspn
Cumin	1 tspn
Chili Powder	¼ tspn
Can of Whole Peeled Tomatoes	28 oz
Eggs	6 large
Salt & Pepper	to taste
Fresh Cilantro, Chopped	small bunch
Parsley, Chopped	small bunch

What is Shakshuka? When my friend introduced me to this dish, I said "Where have you been all of my life". Shakshuka is a classic North African and Middle Eastern dish and one that's eaten for breakfast or any meal of the day. It's made from simple, healthy ingredients and is vegetarian. Shakshuka literally means "a mixture" and the traditional version uses tomatoes, onions and spices as the base with eggs poached on top.

🔥 SERVED HOT

🌙 SAVORY

1 Heat olive oil in a large sauté pan on medium heat. Add the chopped bell pepper and onion and cook for 5 minutes or until the onion becomes translucent.

2 Add garlic, spices and cook for one minute.

3 Pour the can of tomatoes and juice into the pan and break down the tomatoes using a large spoon. Season with salt and pepper and bring the sauce to a simmer.

4 Use a large spoon to make small wells in the sauce and crack the eggs into each well. Cover the pan and cook for 5-8 minutes, or less if you like your eggs less cooked.

5 Garnish with chopped cilantro and parsley.

Split Pea Soup

(50 Minutes)

Very nourishing soup when your immune system is experiencing stress.

🔥 SERVED HOT

🌿 SAVORY

INGREDIENTS:

Coconut Oil	**1** tbl
Chopped Yellow Onions	**2** cups
Sea Salt	
Freshly Ground Black Pepper	
Crushed Red Pepper Flakes	
Chopped Garlic	**1** tbl
Bay Leaf	**1** leaf
Dried Green Split Peas, Picked Over And Rinsed	**1** lb
Vegetable Broth	**8** cups
Almond Milk	**1** cup
Hot Sauce	

1 In a large soup pot over medium-high heat, heat the oil. Add the onions. Season with sea salt, pepper, crushed red pepper. Sauté for 2 minutes. Add the garlic, bay leaf, and split peas and cook, stirring, for 1 minute. Add the broth and bring to a boil, then reduce the heat to medium and simmer, stirring occasionally, for 45 minutes, until the peas are tender. Remove from the heat and let cool slightly. Remove the bay leaf and discard. Add the mixture into the Emulsifying Blender, process until smooth. Add the hot sauce and serve hot.

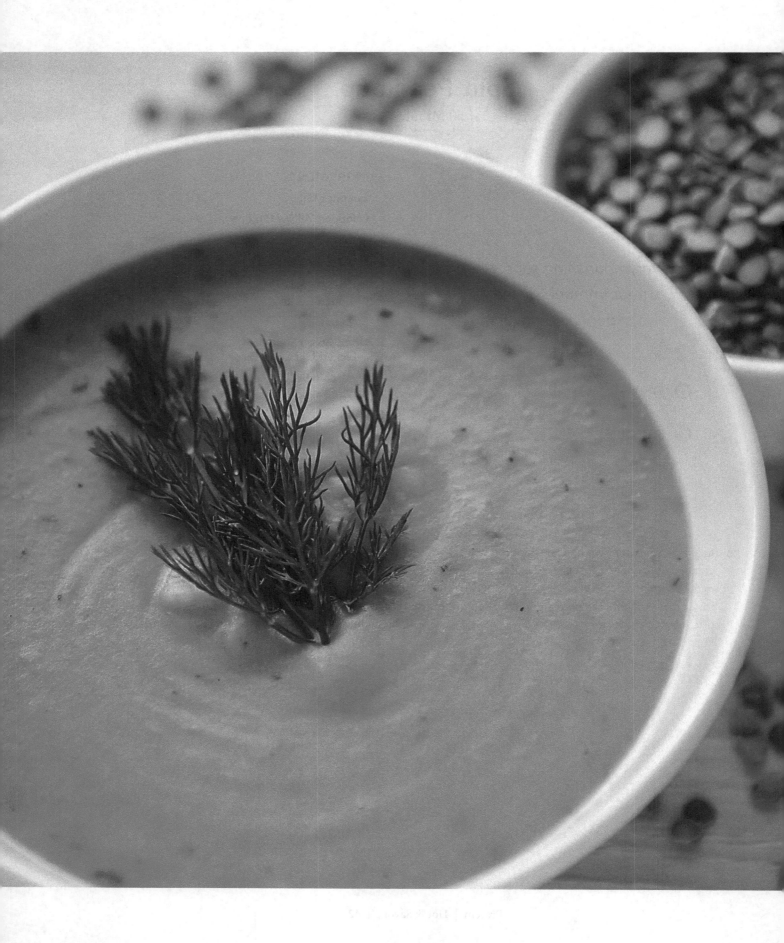

Steak & Edamame Salad

(50 Minutes)

This is a similar recipe from one of my favorite San Diego restaurants, C-Level with a gorgeous view.

🔥 SERVED HOT

🌀 SAVORY

INGREDIENTS:

Grass-Fed Top Round Steak, 3/4 Inch Thick, Trimmed Of Fat	**8** oz
Sea Salt	**½** tspn
Freshly Ground Pepper	**½** tspn
Mixed Asian Greens, Or Mesclun Greens	**4** cups
Snow Peas, Sliced	**1** cup
Red Bell Pepper, Sliced	**1** cup
Shredded Red Cabbage	**½** cup
Cilantro Leaves, Chopped	**½** cup
Shelled Edamame, Thawed	**⅓** cup
Sesame Tamari Vinaigrette	**¼** cup

1 Sprinkle steak with sea salt and pepper. Coat a small nonstick skillet with coconut oil; place over medium heat. Add the steak and cook about 4 minutes per side for medium-rare. Let rest for (at least 5) minutes before slicing.

2 Combine greens, snow peas, bell pepper, cabbage, cilantro, edamame and vinaigrette in a large bowl. Toss to coat. Divide between 2 plates. Top with the steak.

Springing Bowl

(50 Minutes)

INGREDIENTS:

Black Beans, Canned Or Dried (Soak For 12 Hours)	**1** cup
Spinach	**1** cup
Coconut Oil	**1** tbl
Roasted Veggies, Carrots, Beets, Onions, Parsnips, Cauliflower	**2** cups

Roast a bunch of your veggies that need to be eaten and add beans to make a bowl.

◐ SERVED HOT

◐ SAVORY

1 Cook beans in a sauce pan, if canned for a few minutes or if you soaked them, cook for 30 minutes then set aside.

2 Roast Veggies for 45 minutes @ 350 degrees. Drizzle a bit of oil.

3 In a large bowl, place the beans and veggies and then top with Chimichurri or Carrot/Ginger Dressing.

Stuffed Mushrooms

(35 Minutes)

This is a great appetizer or a side dish with your meat of choice.

🔥 SERVED HOT

◐ SAVORY

INGREDIENTS:

Mushroom Caps About 1 Pound Total	**18** large
Reduced-Sodium Chicken Broth	¼ cup
Chopped Shallots	¼ cup
Italian Plum Tomato (Or Other Small Tomato, Diced)	1
Chopped Walnuts	⅓ cup
Goat Cheese	½ cup
Chopped Fresh Tarragon (Or 1 tspn Dried Tarragon)	1 tbl
Sea Salt And Pepper (To Taste)	
Coconut Oil	

1 Preheat oven to 375° F.

2 stems from mushroom caps, leaving an indentation in underside of each cap to hold filling later. Chop stems and set aside. Coat large nonstick skillet with coconut oil vs. nonstick cooking spray and place over medium-high heat. When hot, add whole mushroom caps and cook about 1 minute on each side, until faintly browned. Place mushrooms, stem end up on baking sheet.

3 Return pan to medium heat and add broth. When boiling, add mushroom stems and shallots, and cook until most of liquid has evaporated, 2 to 3 minutes. Scrape mixture into bowl and add tomato, walnuts, goat cheese and tarragon. Stir to combine, then season with sea salt and pepper to taste.

4 Mound walnut mixture among mushroom caps, placing a generous tablespoon in each one. Bake 15 to 18 minutes, until mushrooms are tender but hold their shape.

Tri-Tip with Grilled Veggies

(40 Minutes)

INGREDIENTS:

Tri-Tip Roast	4 lbs
Garlic, Peeled & Very Thinly Sliced	4 cloves
Sea Salt	¼ cup
Black Pepper	⅓ cup
Garlic Salt	¼ cup
Onion	1
Mushrooms	1 cup
Brussels Sprouts	2 cups
Red Pepper	½

Seaside Market in Cardiff, CA is known for their Tri-Tip. We love to grab this hunk of meat for a summer gathering.

 SERVED HOT

 SAVORY

1 Using a sharp knife, cut small slits into the top of the roast. Stuff the slits with slices of garlic.

2 Mix together salt, pepper, and garlic salt. Rub entire mixture all over the tri-tip. Refrigerate at least an hour and up to all day. Take the meat out of the refrigerator about 20 minutes before grilling.

3 Preheat an outdoor grill for high heat. Place the meat directly above the flame for 5 to 10 minutes per side (depending on thickness) to sear the meat and lock in the juices.

4 Turn the grill down to medium heat and continue to cook for another 25 to 30 minutes, trying not to flip it too much. Check for doneness with a meat thermometer. Thermometer should read at least 145° F (63° C) for medium-rare. Let stand, covered loosely with aluminum foil, for 5 minutes before slicing.

5 Place cut veggies in tin foil or roaster: Onion, mushrooms, Brussels sprouts, red peppers, drizzle with olive oil.

Vegetable Frittata

(45 Minutes)

This can be a Combined Meal (organic free range eggs are on the protein side of the tree and potatoes on the starch, if you remove potatoes then it is a Protein Meal).

🔥 SERVED HOT

🌑 SAVORY

Ingredients:

Organic Free Range Eggs	**8** large	
Organic Milk (Optional)	**¾** cup	
Sea Salt	**½** tspn	
Freshly Ground Pepper	**¼** tspn	
Olive Oil	**3** tbl	
Onion Halved & Thinly Sliced	**1** medium	
All-Purpose Potato (7 Ounces)	**1**	
Cut Into 3/8-Inch Cubes (Optional)		
Small Broccoli Florets	**1** cup	
Small Cauliflower Florets	**1** cup	
Spinach	**2** cups	
Fresh Goat Cheese	**5** tbl	

1 Preheat oven to 375° F. Beat organic free range eggs, milk, sea salt, and pepper in medium bowl.

2 Heat oil over medium heat, in medium nonstick (10-inch) sauté pan. Add onions and potatoes and cook until onions are softened, 8 minutes, stirring occasionally.

3 Stir in broccoli, spinach, and cauliflower; cook until vegetables are tender, 10 minutes, stirring occasionally.

4 Reduce heat to low and pour in organic free range egg mixture. Drop small spoonfuls of goat cheese on top. Cook about 2 more minutes on the stove.

5 Transfer to oven and bake 20 to 25 minutes, or until the top is golden brown and the organic free range eggs have just set in the center. Note that if you are using a skillet with a nonmetal handle; wrap it with double-thickness aluminum foil before placing in oven. Remove from oven and slide out of pan onto a cutting board. Cut into wedges and serve warm.

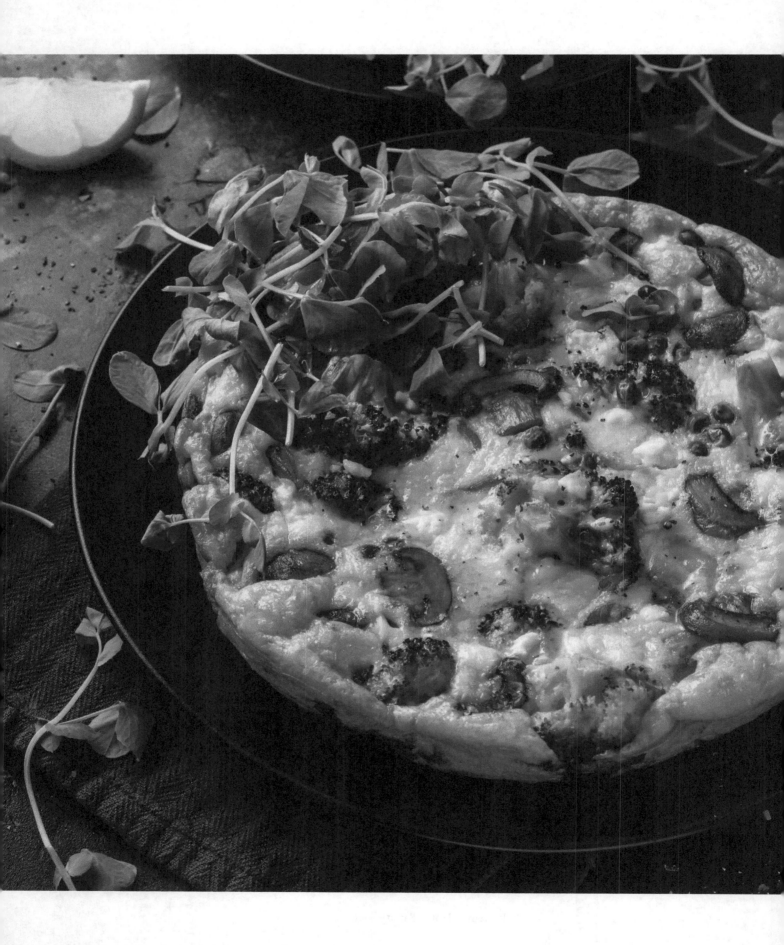

Vegetarian Stuffed Tomatoes

(60 Minutes)

*Another great appetizer or a
colorful side dish.*

🔥 SERVED HOT

🌙 SAVORY

INGREDIENTS:

Round Tomatoes	12	
Sea Salt	1	tbl
Butter	1	tbl
Olive Oil	½	tbl
Sea Salt	1	tspn
Onions	2	large
White Wine	1	cup
Soft Goat's Cheese	12	oz
Organic Free Range Eggs	4	
Fresh Basil Leaves, Chiffonnade	10	
Fresh Black Pepper		
Olive Oil	1	tspn

1 Slice the tops of the tomatoes, removing about 1/4 from the top of each tomato. (These tomato scraps can be saved and used in a salad.) Scoop out the seeds and membranes.

2 Line trays with paper towel. Sea salt the inside of each tomato with a hefty pinch of sea salt. Place them upside down on the paper towel to drain for at least three hours and up to 6 hours.

3 Heat the butter and olive oil in a heavy-bottomed skillet over low heat. Thinly slice the onions and add them to the pan along with the teaspoon of sea salt. Allow to cook, stirring occasionally, until the onions begin to brown and all moisture has evaporated from the pan. Deglaze the pan with some of the white wine. Continue cooking, deglazing with wine as needed, until the onions are caramelized. If the wine is finished, use water. After about 45 minutes, the onions should be deep, mahogany brown.

4 When the tomatoes have drained, preheat the oven to 350° F. In a large mixing bowl, whisk the goat's cheese until it is creamy. Add the organic free range eggs, one by one, whisking after each addition. Add the caramelized onions, basil and black pepper. Whisk to combine.

5 Line a baking dish with parchment paper and place the tomatoes on it. Fill each tomato with an equal amount of the filling. Sprinkle olive oil and parmesan cheese over the top. Bake the tomatoes for about 20 minutes.

Wild Salmon & Creamed Spinach

(22 Minutes)

INGREDIENTS:

Salmon Fillets	**4** (6 oz)
Kosher Salt	
Freshly Ground Black Pepper	
Shredded Mozzarella	½ cup
Frozen Spinach, Defrosted	½ cup
Garlic Powder	¼ tspn
Pinch Red Pepper Flakes	
Grass Fed Butter	2 tspn
Lemon Juice	½ lemon

A satiating protein meal to support your Omega's 3's and creamy texture craving.

🔥 SERVED HOT

🌿 SAVORY

1   Season salmon all over with salt and pepper. In a large bowl, mix mozzarella, spinach, garlic powder, and red pepper flakes.

2   Using a paring knife, slice a slit in each salmon to create a pocket. Stuff pockets with cheese mixture.

3   In a large skillet over medium heat, heat oil. Add salmon skin side down and cook until seared, about 6 minutes, then flip salmon. Add butter and squeeze lemon juice all over. Cook until skin is crispy, another 6 minutes. Serve warm.

Chinese Shrimp & Broccoli

(25 Minutes)

We all crave a hot meal from a Chinese restaurant. Try this recipe to satisfy those taste buds and without the MSG.

🔥 SERVED HOT

🌑 SAVORY

INGREDIENTS:

Uncooked Shrimp	**2** lbs
Coconut Oil	**2** tspn
Onion, Thinly Sliced	**1**
Head Broccoli, Cut Into Small Florets	**1**
Garlic, Minced	**2** cloves
Minced Ginger	**1** tbl
Oranges	**2**
Braggs Liquid Amino Acids	**1** cup
Raw Honey	**1** tbl
Sesame Oil	**1** tbl
Brown Rice Flour	**2** tbl
Water	**¼** cup

1. Peel and vein the shrimp if necessary.

2. In a wok or heavy skillet, heat the coconut oil over high heat. Add the onion. Cook until just beginning to brown, about 5 minutes. Add the broccoli and toss to combine. Cook until the broccoli begins to turn a brighter green, about 3 minutes. Add the garlic and ginger and cook until fragrant, about 1 minute.

3. Add the juice of the oranges, the Braggs sauce, the honey and the sesame oil. Cook, stirring occasionally, until the broccoli is cooked to the desired doneness.

4. Meanwhile, dissolve the brown rice flour in the water.

5. When the broccoli is cooked remove it to a plate. Add the water and cornstarch mixture to the pan, and whisk until you have an even, thick sauce. Add the broccoli back to the pan and add the shrimp. Cook until the shrimp just turn pink, about 3-4 minutes.

Egg Crepes

(5 Minutes)

INGREDIENTS:

Organic Free Range Egg	1
Water	1 tbl
Kosher Salt	1 pinch
Coconut Oil For Cooking	

Great idea for a light breakfast. Top with savory vegetables or sweet almond butter and honey.

🔥 SERVED HOT

🌑 SAVORY

1 Whisk all ingredients together until thoroughly mixed, with organic free range egg beaten but not overly frothy.

2 Heat a bit of coconut oil in a small pan or crepe pan over medium heat. Pour about 2 tablespoons of batter into a thin layer in the pan. Rotate the pan or use a crepe paddle to evenly coat the bottom of your pan.

3 Cook for 2 minutes, or until the crepe's edges begin to pull away from the pan. Flip and cook for another minute.

4 Repeat with remaining batter and serve.

Roasted Organic Chicken with Moroccan Spices

(60 Minutes)

These spices are wonderful to support your taste buds and are warming for your soul.

🔥 SERVED HOT

🍓 SWEET

INGREDIENTS:

Olive Oil	**3** tbl
Fresh Lemon Juice	**3** tbl
Hungarian Sweet Paprika	**2** tbl
Ras-El-Hanout	**1** tbl
Chopped Fresh Mint	**1** tbl
Sea Salt	**1** tbl
Grated Lemon Peel	**2** tspn
Ground Black Pepper	**1** tspn
Garlic, Peeled	**1** clove
Whole Free-Range Organic Chicken (4-3/4 To 5 Pound)	**1**
Whole Lemons, Pierced All Over With Fork	**2** small
Garlic, Unpeeled	**6** Cloves

1   Position rack in center of oven and preheat to 400° F. Blend first 9 ingredients in blender to moist paste.

2   Remove neck, giblets, and excess fat from main cavity of chicken. Rinse chicken inside and out; pat dry with paper towels. Rub 1/3 of spice paste into main cavity and neck cavity, then rub remaining spice paste all over outside of chicken. Place lemons and garlic cloves in main cavity of chicken. Tie legs together. Place chicken on rack in roasting pan. Roast 45 minutes; tent with foil to prevent overbrowning. Continue to roast chicken until instant-read thermometer inserted into thickest part of thigh registers 170° F, about 45 minutes. Transfer chicken to platter; let stand 10 minutes (internal temperature will increase by 5 to 10 degrees).

Thai Chicken Lettuce Wraps

(15 Minutes)

🔥 SERVED WARM

🍓 SWEET

Great meal or appetizer any time of year.

INGREDIENTS:

Rice Vinegar	¼ cup
Olive Oil	¼ cup
Lime Juice	2 tbl
Mayonnaise	2 tbl
(See Mayonnaise Recipe On Page 105)	
Natural Creamy Maranatha Almond Butter	2 tbl
Pure Cane Dark Brown Sugar	1 tbl
Braggs Amino's Soy Sauce	1 tbl
Minced Fresh Ginger Root	2 tspn
Sesame Oil	1 tspn

Thai Chili Sauce	1 tspn
Garlic, Peeled	1 clove
Minced Fresh Cilantro, Divided	½ cup
Dark Meat Chicken	14 oz
Chopped Green Onions	½ cup
Shredded Carrots	½ cup
Sweet Red Pepper, Diced	1 small
Dry Roasted Almond Slivers, Chopped, Divided	¾ cup
Bibb Or Boston Lettuce Leaves	8

1. Combine the first 11 ingredients in Emulsifying Blender until smooth. Stir in 1/4-cup cilantro.

2. In a large bowl, combine the dark-meat chicken, onions, carrots, red pepper, 1/2 cup almond slivers and remaining cilantro. Add dressing and toss to coat.

3. Divide among lettuce leaves; sprinkle with remaining almond slivers. Fold lettuce over filling.

Artichoke & Tuna Salad

(10 Minutes)

A great meal for a quick and healthy lunch on a summer day.

❄ SERVED COLD

🌙 SAVORY

INGREDIENTS:

Cooked Tuna, Flaked	**6** oz
Chopped Canned Artichoke Hearts	**1** cup
Chopped Olives	**½** cup
Lemon Juice	**2** tspn
Olive Oil Based Mayonnaise Or Our Own Mayo Recipe On Page 105	**2** tspn
Chopped Fresh Oregano, Or ½ Teaspoon Dried	**1½** tspn

1 Combine in bowl and serve.

Beet Hummus

(10 Minutes)

INGREDIENTS:

Garlic	**2** cloves
Coriander	**½** tsp
Lemon Juice	**⅓** cup
Tahini	**⅓** cup
Sea Salt	**1** tsp
Cooked Beets: Roast For 45 Minutes.	**8** oz
Chickpeas, Strained & Rinsed	**2** cans
Olive Oil	**¼** cup
Assorted Herbs, Chopped (My Favorite Is Parsley)	**1** tbsp

To spice up your taste buds and try a new flavor of hummus.

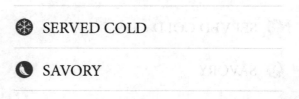 SERVED COLD

SAVORY

1 In a food processor combine the garlic, coriander, lemon juice, tahini and salt.

2 Pulse until the garlic is minced in the lemon juice tahini mixture.

3 Add in the beets and chickpeas and pulse again into an almost smooth paste.

4 Slowly pour in the olive oil with the blades running until the oil is gone and the mixture is finally creamy and smooth.

Borscht

(40 Minutes)

A cooling salad to
help clear and support the colon
and digestive tract.
This salad satisfies all of
your taste buds and cravings
from the Conscious Nutrition
Cravings Book, such as cold,
savory and creamy.

❄ SERVED COLD

🌙 SAVORY

INGREDIENTS:

Beets, Cooked & Peeled	**8** medium
Full Fat Greek Or Goat Yogurt	**¼** cup
Prepared White Horseradish	**1** tspn
Dijon Mustard	**1** tspn
Minced Scallions	**2** tbl
Chopped Fresh Dill	**2** tbl
Lime Juice	**1** tbl

1 Slice, dice or chop the beets to 1/2 inch cubes

2 Place all the remaining ingredients (except the dill) in a serving bowl, add the beets and mix gently but thoroughly.

3 Refrigerate for 1-2 hours.

4 Top with dill and serve.

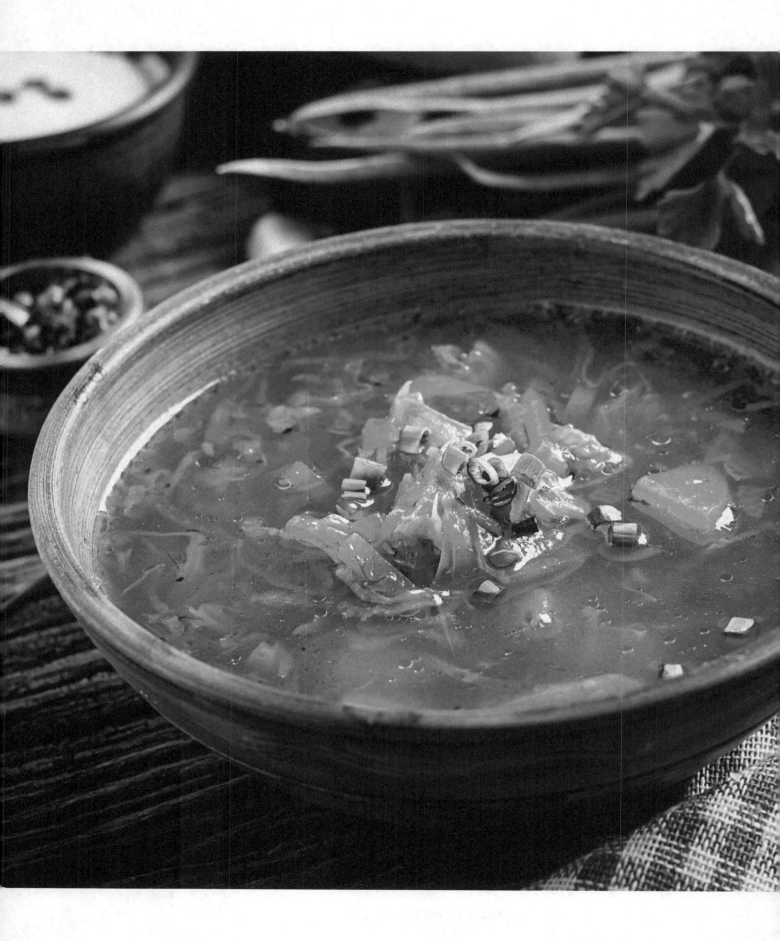

Chicken Salad with Pistachios

(15 Minutes)

Some times hot or warm foods do not sound appealing. This chicken salad is a great meal for those occasions.

❄ SERVED COLD

🌙 SAVORY

INGREDIENTS:

Grilled Chicken, Diced	1 lb
Yellow Bell Peppers, Diced	½ pepper
Fennel Bulbs, Diced	½ large
Red Onion, Soaked In Lemon Juice For 10 Minutes	¼ onion
Pistachios	⅓ cup
Fresh Thyme, Minced	1 tbl
Olive Oil Based Mayonnaise (Recipe In Free Meals) To Taste	
Splash Of Rice Wine Vinegar And/Or Apple Cider Vinegar, Olive Oil	
Kosher Salt & Fresh Ground Pepper (To Taste)	

1 Combine all ingredients in a large bowl and mix well. Season to taste.

Fava Bean Salad with Manchego

(15 Minutes)

Fresh spring bean salad with my favorite cheese!

❄ SERVED COLD

🌙 SAVORY

INGREDIENTS:

Shucked Fresh Fava Beans	4 cups
Fresh Lemon Juice	¼ cup
Minced Garlic	2 tbl
Olive Oil	¼ cup
Salt & Freshly Ground Black Pepper	
Manchego Cheese, Shaved Thinly (Or Asiago Or Romano)	¼ lb
Finely Chopped Flat Leaf Parsley	2 tbl

1 Fill a bowl with ice and water. Bring a large pot of salted water to a boil. Add the fava beans and cook until just tender, 3 to 4 minutes. Drain and shock in ice water. Drain again and remove outer skins. Place the beans in a medium serving bowl. In a small bowl, combine the lemon juice, garlic and olive oil and whisk until blended. Season with salt and pepper to taste. Pour the mixture over the beans and mix well. Add the cheese, sprinkle with the parsley and serve.

Lentil Salad

(7 Minutes for prepared lentils)

INGREDIENTS:

French Green Lentils	**1** cup
Head Radicchio, Sliced Thin & Chopped	**½**
Shallots, Finely Chopped	**3** tbl
Radishes, Sliced Thin & Chopped	**2**
Carrots. Peeled & Grated	**½** cup
Red Wine Vinegar	**1** tbl
Roughly Chopped Parsley & Basil	**3** tbl
Sea Salt & Fresh Ground Pepper	

At your grocery store, look for prepared lentils that are perfect for this meal.

❄ SERVED COLD

◐ SAVORY

1 Place lentils in a medium size saucepan, and cover with about three inches of filtered water and bring to a boil. Reduce to a simmer and cook until just tender about 20-30 minutes, do not overcook or they will become mushy (add more water if necessary). Drain lentils.

2 Toss lentils with red wine vinegar, sea salt and fresh ground pepper. Let sit for 5 minutes. Toss with olive oil, shallots, radicchio, radishes and fresh herbs. Taste and adjust seasoning for flavor. Can be served chilled or room temperature.

Organic Free Range Egg Salad

(25 Minutes)

This is a great meal for either breakfast or lunch. Top on greens for a protein salad meal.

✴ SERVED COLD

◗ SAVORY

INGREDIENTS:

Organic Eggs	**6** large
Make Your Own Mayonnaise (See Our Mayo Recipe On Page 105)	**2** tbl
Organic Whole-Grain Mustard	**1** tbl
Organic Celery, Washed & Chopped	**2** stalks
Organic Dill Pickle, Washed & Chopped	**1** small
Organic Red Onion, Washed & Chopped	**¼** onion
Lemon Juice	**1** tbl
Garlic Powder	**¼** tspn
Sea Salt And Pepper (To Taste)	

1 Place organic free range eggs in a large saucepan and cover with cold water by about an inch. Close the pot tight with a lid.

2 Bring to a boil and let boil for one minute. Cover; remove from heat, and let sit for 8 minutes.

3 Prepare a large bowl with ice water, and after the 8 minutes are over, place the organic free range eggs inside of it and let sit for 3 minutes. Now you can peel the organic free range eggs into a large bowl, and if they're difficult to peel, don't worry – that just means they are very fresh!

4 In the large bowl, add the mayonnaise, mustard, sea salt, pepper, garlic powder and lemon juice. Chop it all together with your fork, but don't mush it up too much — you want there to be chunks of organic free range eggs.

5 Add the onion, celery and pickle. Mix it all together lightly and enjoy!

Options and serving suggestions

Leave out a few of the yolks to make it lighter and feed yolks to your dog!

Add a dollop of sweet pickle relish for a sweet and zesty snap.

Serve organic free range egg salad topped with parsley out of pudding dishes for a light ladies lunch.

Spread on brown rice toast and top with lettuce and tomato for an all-star sandwich. (Combined Meal)

Top rice crackers with the salad, then layer with a small slice of avocado. (Combined Snack)

Add some jalapeno flakes and fresh chopped cilantro and serve with tortilla chips for a little taste of Mexico

Spinach & Lentil Salad

(5 Minutes)

INGREDIENTS:

Spinach Or Mixed Greens	1 cup
Artichoke Hearts	½ cup
Hearts Of Palm	½ cup
Lentils Or Hummus	½ cup
Broccoli	½ cup
Olive Oil	1 tbl
Vinegar	1 tbl
Sea Salt & Pepper (To Taste)	

This is great to make at home or to grab at a conscious salad bar.

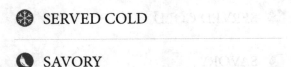

❄ SERVED COLD

🌙 SAVORY

1   Combine vegetables and greens. Mix oil, vinegar, lentils or hummus together in a separate bowl.

2   Combine and toss. The hummus offers a creamier dressing

Arugula Salad

(15 Minutes)

This light salad offers satiety and cleansing properties.

❄ SERVED COLD

🍓 SWEET

SALAD

Organic Mixed Spring Greens	8 cups
Finely Chopped Organic Kale, Chard Or Collards	1 cup
Organic Meyer Lemon, Sectioned Into 8 Slices	1
Organic Herbed Goat Cheese, Sliced	4-6 oz

STRAWBERRY RHUBARB VINAIGRETTE

Organic Rhubarb, Chopped	¼ cup
Frozen Organic Strawberries, Thawed	1 cup
Organic Spring Onions Or Shallots, Chopped	3
Raw Honey	1 tbl
Organic Apple Cider Vinegar Or Fruit Vinegar	⅓ cup
Organic Olive Oil	¾ cup
Organic Mustard	¼ tspn

1. Toss greens in a salad bowl and divide equally onto four plates. Place 2 lemon sections and slices of herbed goat cheese on top of each salad.

2. To make the vinaigrette place rhubarb, strawberries and spring onions in a food processor and blend until smooth. Pour mixture into a bottle or jar through a funnel, add the remaining ingredients, place a cap on the bottle and give it a good shake. Serve the vinaigrette on the side.

Ceviche with Papaya Salsa

(5 Minutes after fish has marinated)

CEVICHE:

Fish About white fish, chopped very small	**2** lbs
Lime Juice	**3** limes
Lemon Juice	**3** lemons
Kosher salt	

PAPAYA SALSA:

Red Onion, **Chopped Very Fine**	**1**
Garlic, Diced	**2** cloves
Papayas, Seeded, **Peeled & Diced**	**2-3**
Red Pepper, Diced	**1**
Jicama, Diced	**½**
Jalapeno, **Chopped Very Fine**	**1**
Roma Tomatoes, **Seeded & Diced**	**2**
Rice Wine Vinegar	**¼** cup
Chili Powder, Coriander, & Black **Pepper To Taste**	
Cilantro (Add Just Before Serving)	
Extra Lime Or Lemon Juice **As Needed For Flavor**	

*Papaya has an enzyme and can be combined with protein.
It is also a great fruit to have as a snack if you are experiencing bloating or headaches.*

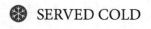 SERVED COLD

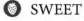 SWEET

Ceviche

1   Combine top two ingredients and put in glass container, refrigerate at least 4 hours.

Papaya Salsa

1   Combine ingredients in an Emulsifying Blender and blend to desired consistency.

Protein Shakes

(10 Minutes)

If you add Protein Powder of your choice, these will be Protein Meals, without Protein, they are Vegan Meals.

❄ SERVED COLD

🍓 SWEET

THE PROTEIN SHAKE

Handful Of Spinach	
Protein Powder	**2** scoops
Unsweetened Almond Milk	
Ice	

BERRY COCONUT SMOOTHIE

Mixed Berries	**1** cup
Coconut Milk	**1** cup
Unsweetened Cocoa Powder	**2** tbl
Honey	**1** tbl

PUMPKIN SMOOTHIE

Pumpkin Puree	**¼** cup
Banana, Fresh Or Frozen	**1**
Coconut Milk	**½** cup
Cinnamon	**1** dash
Honey	**1** tspn
Almond Butter	**1** tbl

The Protein Shake

1 Blend and enjoy!

Berry Coconut Smoothie

1 Blend and enjoy!

Pumpkin Smoothie

1 Combine pumpkin puree, banana, coconut milk, cinnamon, and honey in an Emulsifying Blender. Blend on high until well mixed and smooth. Pour in a glass and garnish with a sprinkle of cinnamon. Enjoy!

Strawberry Coconut Cream Smoothie

(10 Minutes)

INGREDIENTS:

Strawberries	**1** cup
Coconut Cream	**1** cup
Water	**1** cup
Ice	

*To support your sweet tooth along with your inner child
This smoothie aids in digestive health and renewal.*

❄ SERVED COLD

🍓 SWEET

1 Blend and enjoy

Mint Chocolate Chip Smoothie

(10 Minutes)

INGREDIENTS:

Cacao Powder (No Sugar Or Sweeteners Added)	**2** tbl
Fresh Mint	**⅛** cup
Almond Milk	**2** cups
Banana	**1**
Almond Butter	**1** tbl
Ice	

The title says it all!

❄ SERVED COLD

🍓 SWEET

1 Blend and enjoy

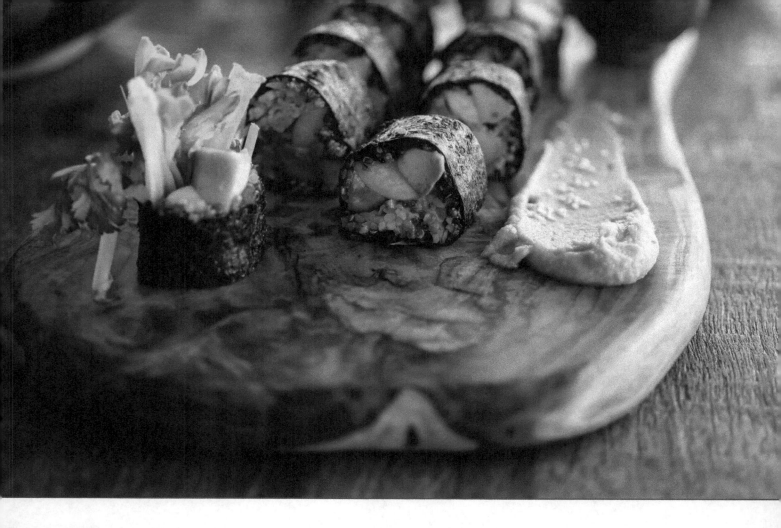

🎃 Starch Meal Recipes

Many diet plans omit starches. However, Conscious Nutrition believes in teaching you HOW to eat. These recipes follow the left side of the tree. Most people tend to combine protein and starches too often. Try experimenting with starches, healthy fats and vegetables. In my practice, I have people who try starch meals at lunch vs. in the evening, and notice more energy and their jeans start to fit better.

Enjoy!

Asparagus with Lemony Fettuccine Noodles

(22 Minutes)

A light pasta dish to support starch cravings.
This combination is one of my favorites to have when you need cozy and comforting.

⬤ SERVED HOT

⬤ SAVORY

INGREDIENTS:

Fettuccine Noodles (Gluten-Free If Desired)	**1**	lb
Asparagus	**1**	bunch
Garlic Minced	**3**	cloves
Lemons 1 Halved & 1 Sliced Into Thin Rounds	**2**	
Shallots Minced	**2**	
White Wine	**½**	cup
Sea Salt	**½**	tspn
Black Pepper	**¼**	tspn
Olive Oil		

1   Bring a large pot of salted water to boil. Add noodles and cook according to package directions. Drain and set aside.

2   Meanwhile, heat a grill or grill pan lightly brushed with olive oil over medium-high heat. Chop the bottom ¼ inch off the ends of the asparagus and compost. Drizzle the spears with olive oil. Squeeze half a lemon over them and then add to the grill. Grill for 4-6 minutes until fork tender. Remove from heat and set aside.

3   Heat a saucepan over medium-low heat. Add 1 tablespoon olive oil and minced shallots. Sauté for 2 minutes. Add garlic and sauté for 2 more minutes. Add white wine, sea salt, and pepper and raise heat to medium until bubbles appear. Simmer for 10 minutes. Add juice from half a lemon. Remove from heat.

4   Add the noodles to the sauce and toss. Add a couple of tablespoons of olive oil if the pasta seems too dry. Top each plate of pasta with grilled asparagus, and lemon slices. Garnish with nutritional yeast if desired. Enjoy!

Bok Choy, Mushroom Quinoa Stir-fry

(35 Minutes)

INGREDIENTS:

Quinoa Cooked	**1**	cup
Bok Choy Rinsed & Patted Dry	**1**	lb
Sliced Mushrooms Crimini Or White	**8**	oz
Garlic Minced	**2**	cloves
Ginger Peeled & Minced	**1**	tbl
Sunflower Oil	**2**	tbl

FOR THE SAUCE:

Low Sodium Tamari Or Bragg's Soy Sauce	**½**	Cup
Organic Chili Sauce	**2**	tbl
Rice Wine Vinegar	**2**	tbl
Sesame Oil	**2**	tspn

A great way to get umami texture without the meat.

 SERVED HOT

 SAVORY

1   Cut the base off of the bok choy. Separate the leaves and then set aside. In a medium bowl, whisk together tamari, chili sauce, rice wine vinegar, and sesame oil. Set aside.

2   Heat oil over medium-low heat. Add garlic and ginger and sauté for 3 minutes. Add mushrooms and raise heat to medium. Stir fry until they are lightly browned. Add bok choy and sauté until lightly wilted for about 1-2 minutes. Add the quinoa and chili sauce and mix until well combined. Remove from heat.

Buckwheat crepes

(30 Minutes)

This non-gluten vegan dish is one of my new favorites. I was taking a break from dairy and eggs so gave this recipe a try and now love them!

🔥 SERVED HOT

🌑 SAVORY

INGREDIENTS:

Buckwheat Flour	1 cup
Backing Powder	1½ tspn
Salt	¼ tspn
Cumin	¼ tspn
Ginger	½ tspn
Pepper	½ tspn
Turmeric	½ tspn
Ginger	½ tspn
Unsweetened Almond or Cashew Milk	13–14 tbl
Apple Cider Vinegar or Lemon Juice	2 tspn

TRY A SWEET OPTION ALSO:

Replace savory spices with the following

Vanilla Extract	1 tspn
Maple Syrup	2 tbl
Cinnamon	1 tspn
Cardamom	½ tspn

Make Sauce

1 Mix the flour, baking powder, salt and spices together in a mixing bowl until well combined.

2 Add the rest of the ingredients and gently fold together until all the flour is wet. If it's a bit clumpy, that's great, do no over mix.

3 Let the batter rest for 8-9 minutes while you heat a non-stick pan or griddle over medium heat.

4 Let cook until bubbles appear all over each pancake and the edges start to look dry and cooked, this should take 3-4 minutes. Flip and cook for 1-2 more minutes.

5 Enjoy right away topped with your favorite pancake toppings or store in the fridge or freezer. Leftovers can be reheated in the toaster or oven.

For savory:

• Sautéed onions and mushrooms, add in middle and fold the pancake like a taco.

For Sweet:

• Top with nut butter, fig jam and maple syrup.

Enchiladas

(50 Minutes)

INGREDIENTS:

Zucchini	2
Summer Squash	2 cups
Onion	1
Corn Tortillas	4

Satisfying different taste buds is supportive in long term success and variety. I recommend to purchase organic and non-GMO corn products.

 SERVED HOT

SAVORY

Make Sauce

1. Sauté chopped onion very low for 10 minutes Do not over brown, but cook slowly

2. Add 1 minced garlic clove, cook for 30 seconds.

3. Add 2 cups water,
   1/2 can diced tomatoes (1 pound size)
   1 pound green chili (frozen chopped)

4. Simmer for 30 minutes

Make Filing

1. Sauté zucchini, summer squash, or combination with onion, and garlic. Mix in diced tomatoes and green chili.

2. Warm Corn tortillas, place on in 9x13 pan add chili sauce and fill with filing. Cover and bake at 375° F for 10 minutes. When bubbly, remove from oven.

Farro & Artichoke Herb Salad

(18 Minutes)

🔥 SERVED HOT

🌑 SAVORY

Give Farro a try to see how your body likes it!

MEAL TYPE:

Starch Meal

INGREDIENTS:

Unsalted Butter	4 tbl
Carrot, Finely Diced	1
Small Celery Root, Peeled & Finely Diced	1
Onion, Finely Diced	1 small
Celery	2 ribs
1 Finely Diced & 1 Thinly Sliced, Plus ½ Cup Celery Leaves	
Bay Leaf	1 leaf

Farro	14 oz
Dry White Wine	1 cup
Low-Sodium Chicken Broth	4 cups
Sea Salt & Freshly Ground Pepper	
Marinated Baby Artichokes Drained And Halved	4 oz ¾ cup
Flat-Leaf Parsley Leaves	½ cup
Snipped Chives	¼ cup
Tarragon Leaves	1 tbl
White Wine Vinegar	1 tspn
Extra-Virgin Olive Oil	1 tbl

1 In a large saucepan, melt 2 tablespoons of the butter. Add the carrot, celery root, onion, diced celery and bay leaf and cook over moderate heat, stirring occasionally, until the vegetables are lightly browned, about 5 minutes. Add the farro and cook, stirring, for 2 minutes. Add the wine and cook, stirring occasionally, until completely absorbed, about 5 minutes. Add half of the broth and cook, stirring occasionally, until completely absorbed, about 12 minutes. Season with salt and pepper. Add the remaining broth and cook, stirring occasionally, until completely absorbed, about 12 minutes longer. Discard the bay leaf. Stir in the grated cheese along with the artichokes and the remaining 2 tablespoons of butter until creamy. Spoon into bowls.

2 In a medium bowl, toss the sliced celery and celery leaves with the parsley, chives and tarragon. Add the vinegar and oil, season with salt and pepper and toss.

Fried Potatoes

(35 Minutes)

INGREDIENTS:

New Potatoes, Sliced In Small Chunks.	**6** medium
Onion, Diced	**½** small
Garlic	**1** tspn
Zucchini, Diced	**1** small
Avocado Oil	**2** tbl
Rosemary	**¼** cup

Sometimes you just need some good ole potatoes. I have a healthy friend who always eats potatoes before she flies to help her feel calm and grounded.

🔥 SERVED HOT

🌿 SAVORY

1 Heat oil, add in garlic and onion.

2 Add in potatoes, cook until half way tender.

3 Add in zucchini and cook taters and zucchini all the way through.

4 Top with rosemary and enjoy!

Gluten Free Porridge

(40 Minutes)

A great breakfast when you want a hot meal. The seasonings and coconut help with blood sugar balance and glycemic index levels versus traditional oatmeals. This oatmeal satisfies all of your taste buds and cravings from the Conscious Nutrition Cravings Book, such as hot, savory, sweet and warming.

INGREDIENTS:

Steel Cut Oatmeal	1 cup
Water	4 cups
Cinnamon	1 tspn
Cardamom	1 tspn
Ground Clove	1 Dash
Nutmeg	1 Dash
Unsweetened Coconut Flakes	⅛ cup
Almond Milk	

🔥 SERVED HOT

🌿 SAVORY

1 Bring 4 cups of water to bowl

2 Slowly add in 1 cup of steel cut oatmeal

3 Stir for 5 minutes as oatmeal thickens

4 Add in all the spices

5 Reduce heat to simmer for 30 minutes

6 Top of with coconut and a splash of almond milk.

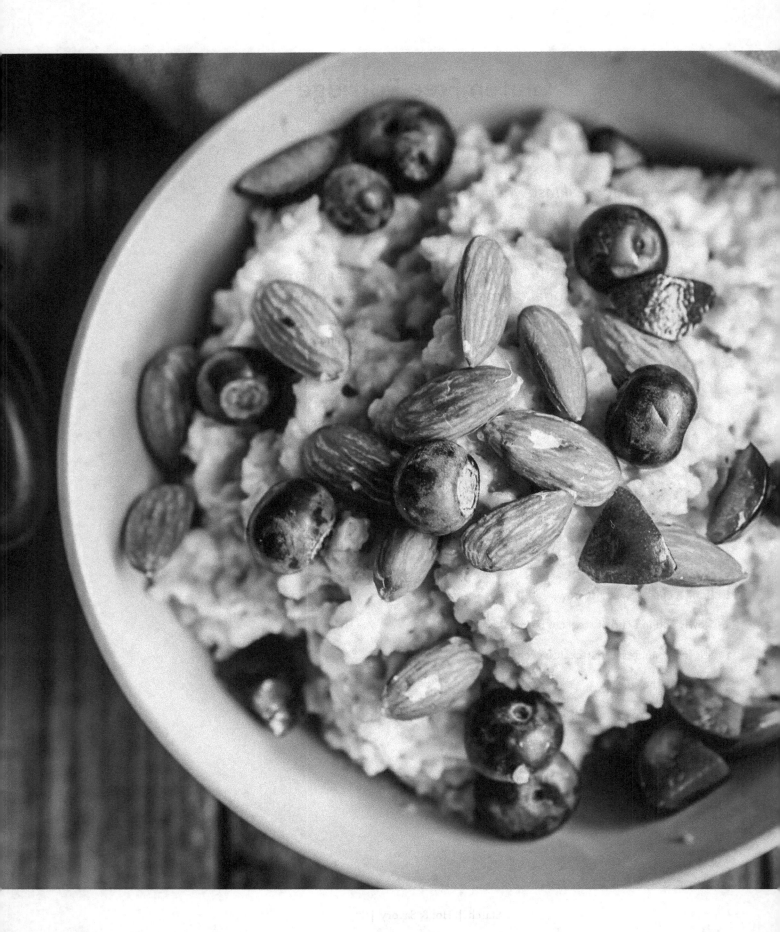

Green Curry De-Light

(22 Minutes)

This warming meal is great for your immune system and you don't have to order out for Thai food! If you are craving meat, add your favorite and leave out the rice to make it a Protein Meal.

⬤ SERVED HOT

⬤ SAVORY

INGREDIENTS:

Coconut Oil	1 1/2 tbl
Green Curry Paste	2 tbl
Coconut Milk	½ cup
Vegetable Broth	½ cup
Bamboo Shoot	4 oz
Snap Peas	1 cup
Chopped Zucchini	1 cup
Spinach	1 cup
Kaffir Lime Leaves Lightly Bruised	5
Thai Basil Leaves	¼ cup
Cooked Basmati Rice	1 cup
Bragg's Soy Sauce	

1   Heat up a pot over medium heat and add the oil. Sauté the green curry paste until aromatic, add the chicken and stir to combine well with the curry paste. Add the coconut milk and water and bring it to a quick boil.

2   Add the bamboo shoots, kaffir lime leaves, zucchini, snap peas and spinach lower the heat to simmer, cover the pot and let simmer for 10 minutes or until the curry slightly thickens.

3   Add the basil leaves. Stir to mix well. Turn off the heat and serve immediately with steamed rice.

Green Pea Veggie Burgers

(50 Minutes)

INGREDIENTS:

Frozen Peas	**2** cups
Garlic, Minced	**2** cloves
Green Bell Pepper, Diced	**1**
Fresh Spinach Leaves, Minced	**½** cup
Cumin	**1** tspn
Coriander Powder	**1** tspn
Tomato Paste	**1** tspn
Brown Rice	**½** cup
Oats	**½** cup
Nut Crumbs (Breadcrumbs Made Out Of Nuts)	**¾** cup
Olive Oil	**¼** cup
Salt & Pepper (To Taste)	

Another great way to have green peas with the texture of a burger.

 SERVED HOT

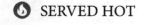 SAVORY

1 Preheat the oven to 400 degrees Fahrenheit.

2 Boil the peas for about 4-5 minutes, drain them and let them cool.

3 Add the peas and all the remaining ingredients into a food processor and blend until it forms into a lump of dough. Add more olive oil to thin it out or more breadcrumbs to thicken it.

4 Form equal-sized patties about the size of your hand. Place them on lightly greased baking parchment paper and flatly slightly with your palm so that they resemble patties.

5 Place in the refrigerator for 30 minutes. Once the patties have set, pop them into the oven and bake for about 25 minutes, keeping an eye on them during the last 5-minute stretch to make sure they don't get too brown.

6 Enjoy them fresh out of the oven or cold, the next day.

Quinoa Stuffed Tomatoes with Dairy Free-Pesto

(42 Minutes)

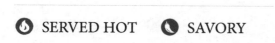

🔥 SERVED HOT ⚫ SAVORY

When you crave Italian food or pizza, EAT THIS! Your body is craving the robust flavors and herbs.

PESTO CREAM

Basil About 2 Cups Lightly Packed Leaves	**2** lg bunches
Olive Oil	¼ cup
Raw Cashews, Soaked	¼ cup
Garlic	1 clove
Nutritional Yeast	1 tspn
Sea Salt & Pepper (To Taste)	

QUINOA FILLING

Olive Oil	**1** tbl
Onion, Diced	1 medium
Fresh Spinach	10 oz
Garlic	3 cloves
Italian Seasoning	½ tspn
Cooked Quinoa	3 cups
Vegan Pesto	6 tbl

TOMATOES

Beefsteak Tomatoes (Seeds And Cores Scooped Out)	**6** lg
Olive Oil	2 tbl
Fresh Basil	

1 Preheat oven to 400 degrees.

2 Pesto: Add all of the pesto ingredients to a high powered blender and blend until smooth and creamy, set aside.

3 Quinoa Filling: In a large sauté pan, sauté the diced onion in olive oil for 5-8 minutes or until translucent. Add the spinach and garlic cloves and cook for 1-2 additional minutes (the spinach should be starting to wilt). Add the cooked quinoa, pesto cream sauce, Italian seasonings, salt, and pepper. Stir to combine.

4 Tomatoes - Cut the top of the tomatoes. Use a   fruit spoon (with a serrated edge) to slip into the tomatoes and scoop out all the seeds and membranes. Set aside.

5 Drizzle a little bit of olive oil in the bottom of a baking dish and spread it around. Place the tomatoes in the baking dish and then drizzle 1 Tbsp of olive oil over the top of the tomatoes. Sprinkle salt & pepper on each tomato.

6 Spoon the pesto quinoa filling into the tomatoes and put the tops back on. Bake for 30 minutes or until the skin starts to blister. Garnish with fresh basil.

Roasted Yams with Quince & Fennel

(50 Minutes)

INGREDIENTS:

Ingredient	Amount
Yams, Diced	2
Fennel Bulbs, Diced	2
Quince, Diced	2
Splash Of Apple Cider	⅛ cup
Olive Oil	¼ cup
Maple Syrup	¼ cup
Kosher Salt	
Browned Butter	
Cinnamon (To Taste)	
Ground Ginger (To Taste)	

This is a great sweet and savory dish to complement both of our favorite cravings. Fennel helps with liver health and inflammation.

◑ SERVED HOT

◑ SAVORY

1 Toss yams, quince, and fennel with remaining ingredients, except browned butter. Roast in preheated 375° F oven for about 45 minutes, until soft and mashy. Brown the butter in a large pan and then add roasted vegetables to the pan. Season with cinnamon, ground ginger to taste, and simmer for another 15 minutes. Stir with wooden spoon, mashing a little to get flavors and ingredients to infuse.

Savory Breakfast Potatoes

(40 Minutes)

Great for camping and when you are more active to burn off the taters!

🔥 SERVED HOT

🌑 SAVORY

INGREDIENTS:

Red Potatoes, Diced Small	**10** medium
Olive Oil	**1** tbl
Garlic Powder	**1** tspn
Sea Salt	**¾** tspn
Red Bell Pepper, Chopped	**½** medium
Dried Rosemary, Crushed	**1** tspn
Basil, Crushed	**1** tspn
Ground Black Pepper	**½** tspn
Fresh Parsley (For Garnish)	**2** tbl

1   Preheat oven to 400° F.

2   Wash and dice potatoes. Mix with oil, herbs and spices. Spread evenly on a cookie sheet.

3   Bake for 30 to 40 minutes, or until desired crispiness. Flip potatoes around every 10 minutes for even browning.

4   Garnish with fresh parsley.

5   Enjoy!

Vegetarian Paella

(45 Minutes)

INGREDIENTS:

Olive Oil	¼ cup
Minced Garlic	5 cloves
Yellow Onion Chopped	1 large
Low Sodium Vegetable Broth	4 cups
Rice (Uncooked)	2 cups
Tomatoes Skinned, Seeded & Chopped	4 medium
Red Bell Pepper, Seeded & Cut Into Thin Strips	1 small
Yellow Bell Pepper, Seeded & Cut Into Thin Strips	1 Small
Green Peas	1 cup
Artichoke Hearts, Tough Outer Leaves Removed & Quartered	2 cups
Lemon	1
Lemon Wedge, To Garnish	

You may need to be extra conscious with timing, so allow yourself not to be rushed making this meal.

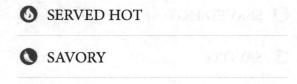 SERVED HOT

SAVORY

1 Heat the oil in a paella pan and sauté the onion and garlic until the onion is tender and translucent. At the same time, heat the broth in a separate saucepan until simmering.

2 Pour the rice into the paella pan and sauté for about 3 minutes.

3 Add the bell peppers and tomatoes and cook for a further 3 minutes.

4 Add the simmering vegetable broth and cook over medium heat for 20 minutes or until almost tender and almost all the liquid has been absorbed.

5 Stir in the peas.

6 Sprinkle the artichoke hearts with a few drops of lemon juice and arrange over the rice in an attractive pattern. Continue cooking until the liquid has been absorbed and the rice is tender.

7 Serve the paella straight from the pan, garnished with lemon wedges.

Vegetable Risotto

(35 Minutes)

I make this on special occasions, it is a crowd pleaser.

🔥 SERVED HOT

🌶 SAVORY

INGREDIENTS:

Lots Of Olive Oil	¼ Cup
Sliced Carrots	½ cup
Sliced Celery	½ cup
Mushrooms Of Your Choice, Sliced	8 oz
Dried Thyme	1 tspn
Arborio Rice	1 cup
Dry White Wine	½ cup
Vegetable Broth	2½ cup
Lemon Juice	¼ cup
Frozen Green Peas	¾ cup
Chopped Parsley	2 tbl
Sea Salt & Black Pepper, (To Taste)	

1 In a heavy bottomed saucepan, heat half of the oil over medium heat. Add the carrots, celery and cook, stirring occasionally, until the celery is tender, about 6-8 minutes. Add the mushrooms and thyme, and sauté until the mushrooms are soft, about 4 minutes more.

2 Add almost the remaining of oil (saving about a tablespoon) and the rice, and, stirring constantly, cook until the rice is evenly coated and sounds like crispy rice cereal in the pan, about 4 minutes. Add the wine, stirring constantly, until all of the liquid is completely absorbed.

3 Begin to ladle the broth into the rice and cook, continuing to stir, until most of the liquid is absorbed. Continue to add the broth in ladleful increments, allowing the liquid to be absorbed before another addition, for about 20 minutes.

4 Add the peas (you can add them frozen) and cook for just about 2-3 minutes, stirring constantly, or until the peas are tender and bright green. Stir in the remaining olive oil, parsley. Add sea salt and pepper to taste and serve immediately.

Vegan Mac-n-Cheese

(45 Minutes)

INGREDIENTS:

Dried Pasta, I love gluten-free penne	**1** lb

For The Vegan Cheese:

Potatoes, Peeled & Chopped	**2** cups
Carrots, Peeled & Chopped	**1** cup
Extra Virgin Olive Oil	**⅓** cup
Unsweetened Plant Milk of Your Choice, I Love Organic Oat Milk	**½** cup
Nutritional Yeast	**½** cup
Lemon Juice	**1** tbl
Salt	**1** tsp
Lemon Juice	**½** tsp
Lemon Juice	**½** tsp

One of my favorite meals on the planet. Even meat and dairy eaters love it.

🔥 SERVED HOT

🌿 SAVORY

---

1. Boil the potatoes and carrots in a large pot for about 20 minutes or until soft.

2. Begin to cook the pasta according to package directions. Drain and set aside.

3. Place potatoes, carrots and the other ingredients for "cheese", in blender to blend smooth.

4. Mix the cooked pasta and the vegan cheese in the pot and if they're both hot, serve immediately.

5. When you reheat it, add a little bit of plant milk if the sauce is too thick.

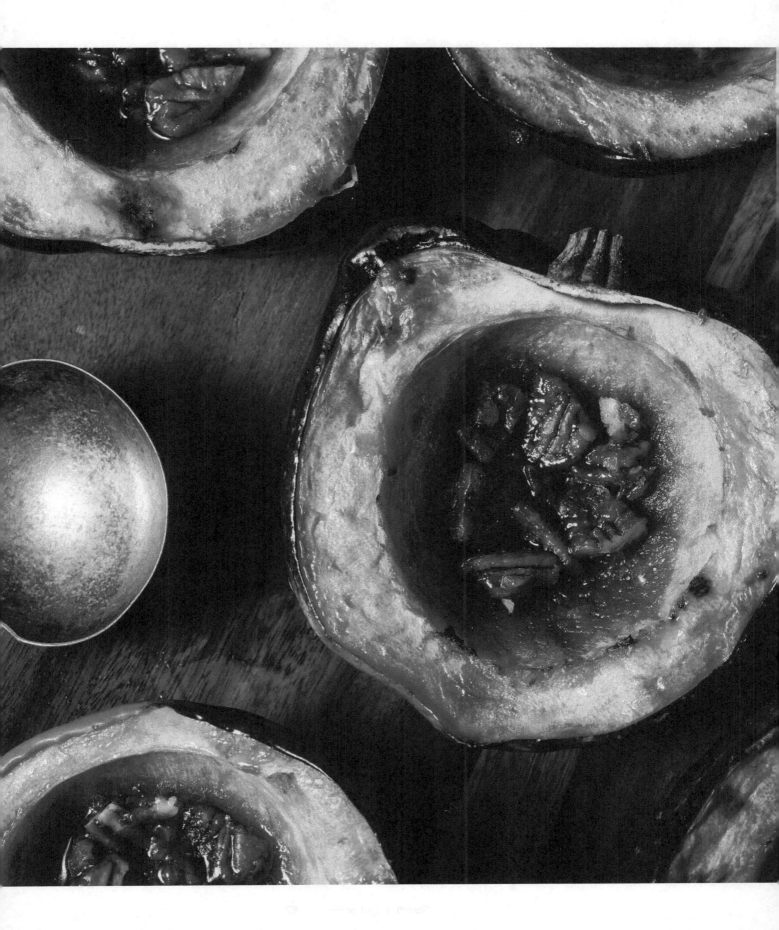

Acorn Squash

(45 Minutes)

INTENTION:

A great light meal or a side dish

INGREDIENTS:

Acorn Squash

Organic Grass Fed Butter Or Ghee

Cinnamon

Drizzle Of Honey For Caramelization

This was my mom and I's go to winter meal back in Nebraska. We would slice an acorn squash in half and bake with butter and cinnamon!

🔥 SERVED HOT

🍓 SWEET

1   Preheat oven to 350 degrees

2   Slice squash in half

3   Add a dollop of butter and sprinkle of cinnamon

4   Bake for 30-45 minutes until it is tender with a fork.

5   Add honey after baking and Enjoy!

Barbecue Portobello Quesadillas

(18 Minutes)

Everyone loves a good quesadilla. When we crave corn often, it is a sign our body's serotonin level is imbalanced between the gut and brain. Be mindful and observe your cravings. Eating more fiber, vegetables, and healthy fat can shift this craving.

🔥 SERVED HOT

🍓 SWEET

INGREDIENTS:

Barbecue Sauce (Without High Fructose Corn Syrup)	½ cup
Tomato Paste	1 tbl
Organic Cider Vinegar	1 tbl
Chipotle Chile In Adobo Sauce, Or ¼ tspn Ground Chipotle Pepper	1 minced
Plus 2 tspn Olive Oil, Divided	1 tbl
Portobello Mushroom Caps Gills Removed, Diced (About 5 Medium),	1 lb
Onion, Finely Diced	1 medium
Sprouted Grain Tortillas Or Corn (8- To 10-Inch)	4
Shredded Organic Raw Cheddar Cheese	¾ cup

1 Combine barbecue sauce, tomato paste, vinegar and chipotle in a medium bowl.

2 Heat 1 tablespoon oil in a large nonstick skillet over medium heat. Add mushrooms and cook, stirring occasionally, for 5 minutes. Add onion and cook, stirring, until the onion and mushrooms are beginning to brown, 5 to 7 minutes. Transfer the vegetables to the bowl with the barbecue sauce; stir to combine. Wipe out the pan.

3 Place tortillas on a work surface. Spread 3 tablespoons cheese on half of each tortilla and top with one-fourth (about 1/2 cup) of the filling. Fold tortillas in half, pressing gently to flatten.

4 Heat 1 teaspoon oil in the pan over medium heat. Add 2 quesadillas and cook, turning once, until golden on both sides, 3 to 4 minutes total. Transfer to a cutting board and tent with foil to keep warm. Repeat with the remaining 1 teaspoon oil and quesadillas. Cut each quesadilla into wedges and serve.

Brown Rice Pasta with Golden Beets & Pine Nuts

(28 Minutes)

INGREDIENTS:

Ingredient	Amount
Pine Nuts	⅓ cup
Olive Oil	4 tbl
Red Onions, Quartered Lengthwise Through Root End, Sliced Crosswise (About 4 Cups)	2 large
Garlic, Minced	3 cloves
Golden Beets With Fresh Healthy Greens; Beets Peeled, Each Cut Into 8 Wedges, Greens Cut Into 1-Inch-Wide Strips (2-Inch-Diameter)	2 bunches
Brown Rice Pasta, Spirals Or Bow Ties	12 oz
Grated Parmesan Cheese Plus Additional For Serving	⅓ cup

Who doesn't crave pasta? This is a fun recipe to try when that craving comes in.

🔥 SERVED HOT

🍓 SWEET

1 Heat heavy large skillet over medium heat. Add pine nuts and stir until lightly toasted, about 3 minutes. Transfer to small bowl. Add 2 tablespoons oil and onions to same skillet and sauté until beginning to soften and turn golden, about 10 minutes. Reduce heat to medium-low and continue to sauté until onions are tender and browned, about 30 minutes longer. Add garlic and stir 2 minutes. Scatter beet greens over onions. Drizzle remaining 2 tablespoons oil over; cover and cook until beet greens are tender, about 5 minutes.

2 Meanwhile, cook beets in large pot of boiling salted water until tender, about 10 minutes. Using slotted spoon, transfer beets to medium bowl. Return water to boil. Add pasta to beet cooking liquid and cook until tender but still firm to bite, stirring occasionally. Drain, reserving 1-cup pasta cooking liquid. Return pasta to pot.

3 Stir onion-greens mixture and beets into pasta. Add pasta cooking liquid by 1/4 cupfuls to moisten. Season with sea salt and coarsely ground black pepper. Stir in 1/3 cup Parmesan cheese. Divide pasta among shallow bowls. Sprinkle with pine nuts. Serve, passing additional cheese.

Creamy Butternut Squash Soup

(50 Minutes)

Squashes are my favorite starch for people to consume. I think Mother Nature is smart and we may need more of these during the winter months when they are abundant.

🔥 SERVED HOT

🍓 SWEET

INGREDIENTS:

Coconut Oil	**2** tbl
Onion, Chopped	**1** small
Celery, Chopped	**1** stalk
Carrot, Chopped	**1** medium
Potatoes, Cubed	**2** medium
Butternut Squash — **Peeled, Seeded, & Cubed**	**1** medium
Container Chicken Stock (32 Fluid Ounce)	**1**
Sea Salt & Freshly Ground **Black Pepper (To Taste)**	

1   Melt coconut oil in a large pot, and cook the onion, celery, carrot, potatoes, and squash 5 minutes, or until lightly browned. Pour in enough of the chicken stock to cover vegetables and bring to a boil. Reduce heat to low, cover pot, and simmer 40 minutes, or until all vegetables are tender. Transfer the soup to an Emulsifying Blender, and blend until smooth. Return to pot and mix in any remaining stock to attain desired consistency. Season with sea salt and pepper.

Healthy Veggie Stir Fry over Quinoa

(15 Minutes)

INGREDIENTS:

Coconut Oil	2	tbl
Dark Sesame Oil, Divided	2	tbl
Garlic, Finely Minced	2	cloves
Fresh Ginger, Crushed	1	tbl
Broccoli, Stems Removed	1	head
Mushrooms, Sliced	1	dozen
Carrots, Peeled & Julienned	3	
Celery, Cut On A Bias	3	stalks
Bok Choy Or Other Greens, Chopped	1	head
Daikon Radish, Peeled & Sliced	1	
Green Onions, Sliced	½	bunch
Braggs Amino Acids To Taste		

This is one of my favorite lunches served warm or cold.

⬤ SERVED HOT

⬤ SWEET

1   Heat oil in a wok or sauté pan over medium-high heat. Add the vegetables and stir. Stir-fry quickly until the vegetables begin to soften. Add the garlic and ginger, then a dash of water, stock, or coconut milk to help cook. Combine well and continue to cook for 5-7 minutes. Dash with Braggs. Serve immediately. Serve stir-fry over quinoa.

Heather's Healthy Pancakes

(15 Minutes)

I love pancakes. Some mornings you just need these and the substance will give you the energy you need for the day.

🔥 SERVED HOT

🍓 SWEET

INGREDIENTS:

Brown Rice Flour	**2** cups
Baking Soda	**½** tbl
Sea Salt	**1** tspn
Cinnamon	**1** tspn
Honey	**1** tbl
Organic Free Range Eggs	**3**
Ripe Banana	**1**
Rice Or Almond Milk,	**1¾** cups
(For More Richness Add Coconut Milk)	

1 Heat and oil frying pan with coconut oil on the stove to about 3.5 or halfway between low and medium. Mix wet ingredients together with mashed banana. Add dry ingredients, mixing well. Pour desired amount of batter (more for bigger pancakes, less for smaller) into warmed pan. Let cook for approximately 3-5 minutes or until you can easy stick your spatula underneath the pancake to fill it over. Cook another 2-3 minutes. Repeat for remaining batter.

2 Try topping with almond butter, ghee, maple syrup, honey, and/or fresh fruit.

3 Enjoy!

Oatmeal with Nut Milk & Almond Butter

(15 Minutes)

INGREDIENTS:

Uncooked Gluten-Free Oatmeal (Or Quinoa Flakes)	½ cup
Almond Butter	1 tbl
Nut Milk	¼ cup
Cinnamon	

I see people who eat the same breakfast often, mostly cereals and oatmeal. I recommend variety and rotation. Pay attention to your sugar cravings two hours after you eat oatmeal and later in the day. If so, eat oatmeal less often.

⬤ SERVED HOT

⬤ SWEET

1 Cook oatmeal or quinoa flakes as directed. Melt in almond butter and top with nut milk and cinnamon.

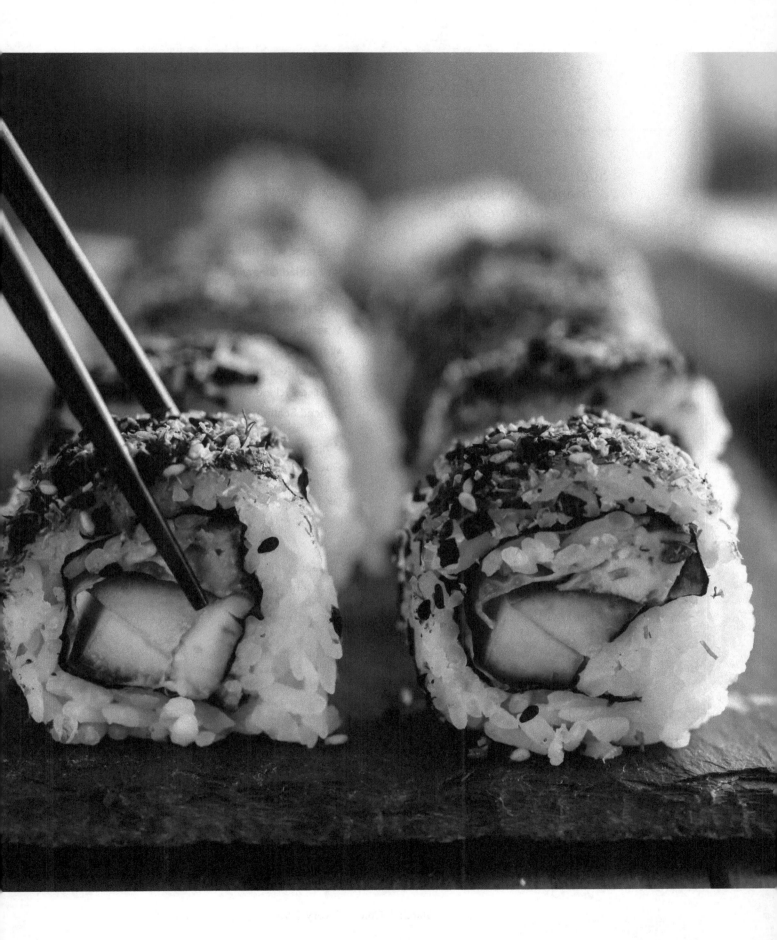

Make Your Own Sushi

(35 Minutes)

Such a fun meal to make with friends, Add fish and it's a Combined Meal

❄ SERVED COLD   ☾ SAVORY

INGREDIENTS:

Sushi Rice	1¼ lb (2 ¾ Cups)
Water	3 cups
Mirin, Plus Additional For Moistening Nori	¼ cup
Nori	5 sheets (1 Package)
Wasabi Powder, Mixed With 2 Teaspoons Water	4 tspn
Small-Diced Red Onion	½ cup
Carrot, Julienned	1
Red Bell Pepper, Julienned	1
Yellow Bell Pepper, Julienned	1
Scallion, Julienned (Green Part Only)	
Hothouse Cucumber,	
Seeded And Julienned	1
Jar Pickled Ginger	1 (10-oz)

SUSHI DIPPING SAUCE

Wasabi Powder	½ tspn
Water	¼ tspn
Crushed Red Pepper Flakes	½ tspn
Minced Pickled Ginger	1 tspn
Minced Scallion (Green Part Only)	1 tspn
White Wine Vinegar	¼ cup
Good Braggs Liquid Aminos	3 tbl
Dark Sesame Oil	½ tspn

1. Place the rice in a strainer and rinse under cold running water until the water is fairly clear, about 5 minutes. Shake the water out and allow the rice to dry in the strainer for 15 minutes.

2. Put the rice in a pot with exactly 3 cups of water and cook covered over high heat until it starts to foam, about 5 minutes. Reduce the heat to low and cook until tender, about 15 minutes. Turn off the heat and sprinkle with 1/4 cup mirin. Replace the lid and allow the rice to steam for 15 minutes. Place in a bowl and cool to room temperature.

3. To prepare the sushi, place a bamboo sushi roller flat on a table with the bamboo reeds horizontal to you. Sprinkle lightly with water. Place 1 nori sheet on top, smooth side down, and moisten lightly with mirin. With damp hands, press 1-1/4 cups rice flat on top of the nori, leaving 1-1/2 inch edges on the top and bottom, but pressing all the way to the sides. Make sure the rice is pressed even and smooth.

4. Spread 1/4 teaspoon of wasabi paste in a horizontal stripe near the lower edge of the rice. Over the wasabi, lightly sprinkle the red onions in a horizontal stripe. Place strips of carrots in a horizontal stripe, on top of the wasabi and onions, and follow by piling the red and yellow peppers, scallions, and cucumbers on top, making a tight, straight bundle of vegetables. Place 1 layer of pickled ginger slices on top.

5. To roll the sushi, pick up the near edge of the bamboo roller and hold it with the nori, then pull them up and over the vegetable bundle until the nori reaches the rice on the other side. Press the roller to make a round bundle, then roll the bundle to the far edge of the nori and press again to make a round bundle. To serve, slice off the ends with a very sharp knife and slice each roll into 8 equal pieces. Then dip into sauces.

Gluten Free Granola

(45 Minutes)

I tend to see people over consume breads, cereals, and grains. It isn't that you can never have these foods again, however when you eat these foods and your body was in dire need of proteins, vegetables and fat, then your body is deprived until it receives these nutrients.

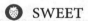 SERVED COLD

🍓 SWEET

INGREDIENTS:

Old Fashioned Gluten-Free Oats	**3** cups
Soaked Coarsely-Chopped Raw Almonds	**1** cup
Shredded Coconut	**½** cup
Packed Brown Sugar	**3** tbl
Ground Cinnamon	**1** tspn
Raw Cocoa	**1** tbl
Ginger	**½** tspn
Sea Salt	**½** tspn
Maple Syrup	**⅓** cup
Olive Oil	**2** tbl
Assorted Dried Fruit Like Goji Berries, Blueberries, Cranberries, or Strawberries	**1** cup

1 Preheat oven to 300° F. Line a baking sheet with a reusable silicone pad or parchment paper (if you don't have a silicone pad).

2 Stir together the first 8 ingredients together in a large bowl. Meanwhile in a small pan over low heat, stir together honey and oil until combined. Pour Maple Syrup and oil mixture over oat mixture and stir to combine.

3 Pour granola mixture out onto lined baking sheet and spread out into an even layer. Bake until golden brown about 40 minutes. Check every 10 minutes to stir and rotate pan. When done, remove cool and pour back into bowl. Stir in dried fruit until combined. Store in an airtight container.

Quinoa & Beet Salad

(55 Minutes)

INGREDIENTS:
list

High quality fiber and heaps of flavor...

INGREDIENTS:

Quinoa	1¼ cups
Sea Salt, Plus More For Dressing	1⅛ tspn
Beets, Trimmed	4 medium
Balsamic Vinegar	2 tbl
Lemon Juice	1 tbl

❄ SERVED COLD   🌙 SWEET

Freshly Ground Pepper, For Dressing	
Extra-Virgin Olive Oil	3 tbl
Seedless Cucumber, Chopped	½ large
Yellow Cherry Tomatoes, Halved	1 pint
Green Beans, Blanched & Cut Into 1-Inch Pieces	1 cup
Chopped Flat-Leaf Parsley	½ cup

💧 SERVED HOT

💧 SAVORY

1 Rinse quinoa thoroughly. Place in a medium saucepan with 2-1/2 cups water. Add 1/8 teaspoon sea salt; bring to a boil. Reduce to a simmer and cover. Cook until quinoa is tender, 12 to 15 minutes. Remove from heat; let stand 10 minutes. Transfer to a bowl. Cover and refrigerate about 2 hours.

2 Meanwhile, place beets in a large saucepan; cover with cold water (by about an inch). Add 1 teaspoon sea salt; bring to a simmer. Cook until beets are tender when pierced with a paring knife, 35 to 45 minutes. Drain; cover with cold water. Let sit until cool enough to handle. Peel and cut into 1/2-inch cubes.

3 In a small bowl, mix vinegar, lemon juice and sea salt and pepper to taste. Slowly whisk in oil. In a large bowl, combine quinoa, beets, cucumber, tomatoes, green beans and parsley. Toss in dressing to serve.

Pumpkin Smoothie

A super supportive smoothie to help with sugar cravings and sustain your energy.

This smoothie is one of my favorites. Fall and winter are the perfect time of year to bring this back in to rotation.

❄ SERVED COLD

🍓 SWEET

INGREDIENTS:

Canned organic pumpkin	½ cup
Almond Milk	1½ cups
Cinnamon	1 tsp
Nutmeg	1 tsp
Spinach	1 cup
Hemp seeds	2 tbl
Ice	

1 Blend and enjoy!

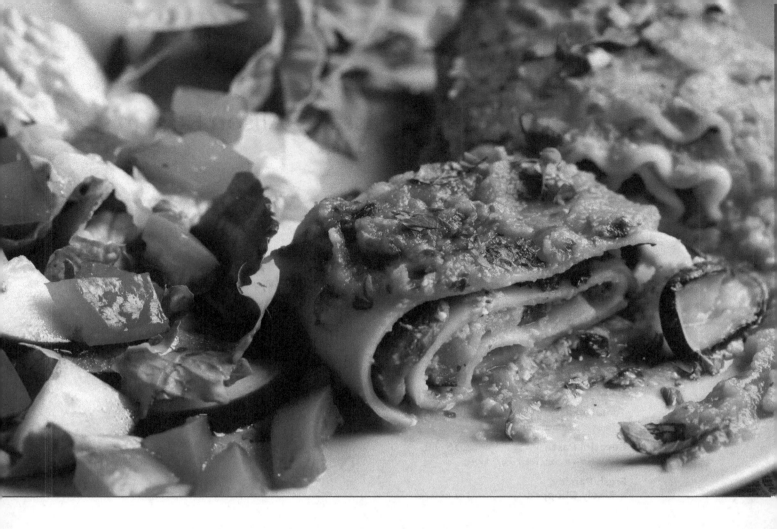

© Combined Meal Recipes

These recipes integrate both sides of the Food Tree. Incorporate when you are feeling great and closest to your health goals. Try having every other day to improve your digestion and notice if you experience more energy.

Enjoy!

Anchovy/Shallot Pasta by Alison Roman's

(35 Minutes)

INGREDIENTS:

Olive Oil	¼ cup
Large Shallots, Sliced Very Thin	6
Garlic Cloves Finely Chopped	6
Salt & Freshly Ground Pepper	to taste
Red Pepper Flakes	1 tspn
Anchovy Filets, drained, but not rinsed.	2 oz can
Tomato Paste (or 4.5 oz tube tomato paste)	6 oz can
Bucatini Pasta (with reserved pasta water...don't forget!)	16 oz pkg
Fresh Parsley, Finely Chopped	1 sm bunch

I saw this dish being made during our COVID times. This woman was teaching Stephen Colbert this recipe and I was HOOKED! It has been a staple in my diet from then on!

🔥 SERVED HOT

🌙 SAVORY

1   Heat olive oil in a heavy dutch oven over medium-high heat. Add the shallots and the garlic and season with salt and pepper. Cook, stirring occasionally until the shallots have softened with golden brown edges. This takes about 20 minutes

2   Add red-pepper flakes and anchovies drained and straight from the can. No need to chop them. They will dissolve when they're cooked. Stir to combine the anchovies with the shallots, about 2 minutes.

3   Add tomato paste and season with salt and pepper. Cook, stirring constantly to prevent any scorching, until the tomato paste has started to cook in the oil a bit, caramelizing at the edges, and turning from bright red to a deeper rusty, brick color, about 2 minutes

4   Remove the pot from the heat and transfer about half of the sauce into a jar, leaving the rest behind. (These are your leftovers that you can use for a future dish).

5   Fill another large pot with salted water and bring to a boil. Cook pasta of your choice, and follow the package instructions or until very al-dente. Save a cup of pasta water when draining. Transfer the cooked pasta to Dutch oven with the remaining shallot mixture and one cup of pasta water. Cook over medium-high heat, tossing the pasta with the shallot mixture to coat each piece of pasta, use a wooden spoon to scape up any bits at the bottom until the pasta is a thick sauce and is reduced and is sticky, but not saucy, 3 to 5 minutes. Divide pasta into bowls or one large serving bowl and top with a little parmesan cheese (optional but I don't think it needs it) and the fresh parsley.

Chardonnay Scallops & Bok Choy with Rice

(38 Minutes)

*This is one of
my personal favorites.*

🔥 SERVED HOT   🌙 SAVORY

POACHED SCALLOPS

Sea Scallops	12	large
Baby Bok Choy	4	heads
Chardonnay Wine	1½	cups
Vegetable Broth	1½	cups
Black Peppercorns	3	whole
Fresh Parsley	3	sprigs
Fresh Dill	3	sprigs
Lemon, Quartered	1	small
Organic, Unsalted Butter	1	tbl
Fresh Dill, Chopped For Garnish		

JASMINE RICE

Chicken Broth	2	cups
Jasmine Rice	1½	cups
Bay Leaf	1	leaf

Jasmine Rice:

1. Bring chicken broth to a boil in a medium saucepan. Stir in rice and bay leaf. Reduce heat to low, cover and cook until rice is tender, about 20 minutes. Remove from heat and let rest for 5 minutes before removing lid. Discard the bay leaf before serving.

Poached Scallops:

1. Find small lobed foot on each scallop and remove before cooking. Trim root end on each head of baby bok choy, slice in half and rinse well to remove any grit.

2. In a large sauté pan, combine wine, broth and peppercorns.

3. Bring to a simmer and lower heat until surface of liquid is barely bubbling. Add parsley and dill. Squeeze lemon wedges into pan and add rinds to liquid. Arrange scallops evenly in pan. Liquid should come just to top of scallops. Poach for 5 minutes, until scallops are firm and opaque in the center. Transfer to a platter and cover to keep warm.

4. Now add bok choy to poaching liquid. Cook for 2 minutes or until just tender and transfer to platter with scallops. Cover to keep warm. Using a slotted spoon, remove lemon rinds, herbs and peppercorns from pan and discard. Increase heat to medium and bring liquid to a rapid simmer. Cook uncovered until reduced by half, about 8 minutes.

5. Take from heat and add butter. Swirl pan until butter melts.

6. To serve, arrange rice, bok choy and scallops on a plate.

7. Drizzle poaching liquid over plates and serve hot.

8. Garnish with the fresh chopped dill.

Chicken Enchiladas

(38 Minutes)

We crave a variety of flavors and textures, it is best to rotate them in to prevent food fatigue. A great weekend meal to satisfy the cozy feeling of staying in with a good hot meal.

🔥 SERVED HOT   🌿 SAVORY

INGREDIENTS:

Tomatillos, Outer Shell Removed	1 lb
Tomatoes, Halved	½ lb
Red Bell Pepper, Seeded & Sliced	1
Onion, Sliced	1
Garlic	2 cloves
Olive Oil	
Lime Juice	2-3 limes
Cilantro	

Organic Corn Tortillas	1 package
Coconut Oil	
Chicken, Roasted With Olive Oil, Sea Salt, Pepper (If Vegetarian, Use Diced Vegetables Like Red Pepper & Zucchini Or Butternut Squash, Roasted)	1 lb
Black Beans	1 can
Avocado	
Sea Salt & Pepper (To Taste)	
Cumin	

1 Roast tomatillos and tomatoes with olive oil and sea salt in 400° F oven until browning. Caramelize onions and green bell pepper in olive oil in skillet on the stove. When soft and golden, add 2 smashed garlic cloves. Cook a few minutes, and then remove from heat. When tomatillos and tomatoes are ready, put in Emulsifying Blender with caramelized onion, bell pepper, and garlic, lime juice, cilantro.

2 Lightly fry tortillas in Coconut oil.

3 Combine chopped roasted chicken and black beans in a bowl. Season to taste with sea salt, pepper, and cumin. Pour about a half-cup of sauce in bottom of baking pan and spread evenly. Roll each tortilla with chicken mixture, lining them up tightly in the baking pan. When they fill the pan, cover in sauce generously, and then top with remaining cheese. Bake at 375° F for about 20 minutes. Remove and serve with sliced avocado, chopped romaine, and chopped tomato.

Coconut Milk Clam Chowder

(40 Minutes)

It still has the butter, but less dairy to help with congestion of lactose in this favorite soup recipe.

◐ SERVED HOT

◐ SAVORY

INGREDIENTS:

Canned Whole Baby Clams (Save The Juice)	**10** oz
Water (Or Vegetable Stock)	**2** cups
Organic Butter	**4** tbl
Chopped Onion	**1** cup
Celery Stalk, Chopped	**1** large
Tomato Paste	**1** tbl
Coconut Milk	**1¼** cups
Red Potatoes, Chopped	**4** small
Dried Thyme	**½** tspn
Sea Salt & Pepper (To Taste)	

1   Boil 2 cups of water in a small pot and add the clams. Save the juice from the can to use for later. Allow to cook for at least 30 minutes with the lid until the clams are soft. Remove from heat and set aside.

2   In a large pot over medium-high heat add the butter, celery, and onion. When the onion begins to turn translucent, add tomato paste and mix until evenly combined. Cook for another two minutes.

3   Add reserved clam juice and coconut milk to the tomato paste mixture and bring to a boil. Once boiling, add the clams (and the water they boiled in), red potatoes, sea salt, pepper, and dried thyme. Simmer until the potato is soft throughout and the soup has reached desired thickness — about 15 minutes.

Fish Stew

(28 Minutes)

INGREDIENTS:

Sweet Potato	**1**
Kale	**4** leaves
Olive Oil	**1** tbl
Garlic, Minced	**1** clove
Zucchini	**1**
Sea Salt (Or To Taste)	**1** tspn
Lime Zest	**1** tspn
Chili Flakes	**¼** tspn
Leek	**1** large (or 2 smaller)
Mahi-Mahi Fillet, Cut Into Bite-Size Pieces	**1** lb
Coconut Milk	**1½** cups
Lime Juice	**1** tbl
Fresh Cilantro	**1** handful

Great meal to make a big pot of and share with your friends.

○ SERVED HOT

○ SAVORY

1 Peel and dice the sweet potato. Cut leek into diagonal slices and rinse. Chop the kale leaves.

2 Heat olive oil in saucepan and sauté garlic for a few seconds. Add the chopped sweet potato, zucchini, sea salt, lime zest and chili flakes, and continue to sauté for a couple of minutes.

3 Add about half a cup of water to the veggies and bring to a boil. Cover pot and simmer for about 5 minutes, then add the leek and continue to simmer for 5 minutes.

4 Add the fish and coconut milk, and simmer until the fish is almost cooked through, about 3 to 5 minutes. (You can add an extra half-cup of coconut milk or water if you prefer a more soupy consistency.) Add the chopped kale and continue to simmer for 2 to 3 minutes.

5 Serve in bowls, drizzled with lime juice and sprinkled with chopped cilantro.

Gluten Free Bean Cakes

(12 Minutes)

*Great alternative to a
veggie burger.*

🔥 SERVED HOT

🌶 SAVORY

INGREDIENTS:

Chickpeas, Drained	1 can
Mary's Gone Crackers Or Nut Thins	1 cup
Zucchini, Chopped	1
Small Red Onion	1
Organic Free Range Egg	1
Sea Salt	1 tspn
Olive Oil	¼ cup
Goat's Milk Yogurt	1 cup
Lettuce	8 leaves
Fresh Mint Leaves	1 cup

1 Blend chickpeas, Mary's Gone Crackers, zucchini, onion, organic free range egg, and sea salt in emulsifying blender.

2 Heat olive oil in pan over medium heat. Form into patties and cook until golden brown 2-4 minutes on each side.

3 Top with yogurt and mint on bed of lettuce.

Grandma Kloppel's Tater Tot Casserole

(45 Minutes)

INGREDIENTS:

Grass Fed Beef	**1** lb
Onion, Diced	**1** medium
Organic Cream Of Mushroom Soup	**1** can
Green Beans	**1** cup
Potatoes, Sliced	**3** medium
Coconut Oil	**1** tbl
Sea Salt & Pepper (To Taste)	

My great grandma brought this comfort dish to almost every family holiday!

⚫ SERVED HOT

⚫ SAVORY

1   Preheat oven to 350° F.

2   Heat oil and add in onion.

3   Add in beef and cook half way through, add sea salt and pepper.

4   Place green beans and soup into a casserole dish. Add in beef and onions.

5   Place the potatoes on top of mixture and bake for 30 minutes.

Kitchari

(45 Minutes)

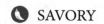

🔥 SERVED HOT   ⚫ SAVORY

An amazing cleansing meal that we use for the Conscious Nutrition RESET program to support liver health.

INGREDIENTS:

Split Yellow Mung Beans	½ cup		Coriander Powder	1½ tspn
White Basmati Rice	½ cup		Ginger Root Freshly Minced	1 tbl
Coconut Oil	2 tbl		Turmeric Powder	½ tspn
Kombu	1 inch stick		Fenugreek Seeds	½ tspn
Homemade Vegetable Stock Or Water	4 cups		Black Mustard Seeds	¼ tspn
Coconut Cream	2 tbl		Any Mixed Vegetables: My Favorite Are Onion, Zucchini, Broccoli & Spinach.	2 cups
Cumin Seeds	1½ tspn		Ghee	2 tbl
Fennel Seeds	1½ tspn		Sea Salt	to taste

1 The night before (24 hours earlier), soak mung beans in ample filtered water.

2 When you're ready to cook, drain the mung beans and rinse under running water. Place rice in a sieve and rinse till the water runs clear. Prepare vegetables by peeling and chopping them up, then set aside.

3 Heat coconut oil over medium heat, in a heavy-bottomed pot. Add cumin, fennel, fenugreek, and black mustard seeds and cook for a few minutes to release aromatics, and until the mustard seeds have popped. Add the rest of the spices and stir to combine.

4 Add a cup of vegetable stock, followed by mung beans, kombu, coconut cream, rice and vegetables, then add the rest of the stock (or water).

5 Cover and bring to a boil, then reduce to a low heat. Simmer for about 40 minutes. Check the pot periodically as the rice swells and may stick to the bottom. Add more water if you want a soupier consistency, and simmer longer to get a thicker stew.

6 Serve and top with ghee!

Mac & Cheese

(35 Minutes)

INGREDIENTS:

Uncooked Elbow Macaroni – Gluten Free	2 cups
Organic Grass-Fed Butter	1 tbl
Yellow Onion	1 small
Butternut Squash (4-5 Cups Cubed)	1 small
Vegetable Broth	5 cups
Unsweetened Cashew Milk	¾ cup
Salt	1 tspn
Shredded Cheese – I Like Gruyère But Any Kind Will Work	⅔ cup
Parsley For Topping	
Salt & Pepper (To Taste)	

Intention:
TOTALLY a comfort meal :)
Enjoy!

🔥 **SERVED HOT**

🌙 **SAVORY**

1 Cook the macaroni according to package directions. Drain and set aside. Heat the butter in a large skillet over medium-low heat. Cut the onion into thin rings and add to the butter in the pan, sautéing over low heat until fragrant and golden, about 15 minutes.

2 Meanwhile, remove the skin and the seeds from the squash. Cut the flesh into small cubes. Bring the broth to a boil and add the squash. Cook for 5-7 minutes or until fork tender. Drain, reserving 1/2 cup broth, and transfer squash to the blender. Add the onions, milk, salt, and reserved broth and puree until completely smooth and creamy. This should yield about 4 cups sauce.

3 Pour the pureed sauce over the cooked noodles and add the shredded cheese. Stir to melt the cheese; add milk to adjust consistency as needed. Serve with parsley, salt, and pepper to taste.

Lasagna (Gluten Free)

(90 Minutes)

Lasagna and Italian Food offers so many flavors and we deserve them!

🔥 **SERVED HOT**   🌙 **SAVORY**

INGREDIENTS:

10 oz Boxes Of Gluten Free Lasagna Noodles (Brown Rice Lasagna Noodles)	2
Finely Chopped Red Onions	1 cup
Finely Minced Cloves Garlic	4
Olive Oil	4 tbl
Sea Salt	1 tbl
Lean Ground Grass-Fed Beef Or Ground Turkey (Optional)	2 lbs
Gluten Free Italian Seasoning Blend	2 tbl
Coarsely Ground	

Fennel Seeds	1 tbl
Marinara Sauce	30 oz
Soft Goat Cheese	½ lb
Ricotta Cheese	1 lb
Freshly Grated Organic Parmesan Cheese	½ cup
Lightly Beaten Organic Free Range Eggs	2
Finely Chopped Fresh Basil	½ cup
Finely Chopped Fresh Italian Parsley	¼ cup
Finely Chopped Fresh Oregano Leaves	¼ cup
Shredded Organic Mozzarella Cheese	1 lb

1   Preheat oven to 350° F.

2   Fill a large stockpot 2/3rds full with cold water. Add 1 teaspoon of sea salt and 1 tablespoon of olive oil, cover with a lid, and bring to a rolling boil. Add 14 gluten free lasagna noodles and boil for 13-14 minutes. (Do not overcook the noodles. They will continue to cook once the lasagna is baked in the oven). Drain and rinse the noodles in cold water. Pour 1 tablespoon of olive oil on the noodles and coat. This will prevent the noodles from sticking together as they cool.

3   Add onions, garlic and 3 tablespoons of olive oil to a large skillet. Sauté for two minutes. Add the ground beef, 1-teaspoon sea salt and brown over medium heat, stirring occasionally, until thoroughly cooked. Pour the canned pizza sauce over the beef mixture, add 1 tablespoon of the Italian seasonings and the entire fennel, stir to mix and simmer for 10 minutes. Stir occasionally to prevent burning.

4   In a medium size mixing bowl, blend goat cheese, ricotta cheese, Parmesan cheese, organic free range eggs, fresh basil, Italian parsley, fresh oregano, 1 teaspoon sea salt, and fresh cracked pepper.

5   Assemble lasagna: Spread 1 cup of the meat sauce mixture in the bottom of the baking dish. Overlap the edges of 4 lasagna noodles on top of the sauce. Evenly spread 1 cup of meat sauce over the noodles. Spread 1 cup of the cheese/herb mixture over meat sauce. Evenly sprinkle about 2 cups of shredded cheeses over this layer. Repeat layers (lasagna noodles/meat sauce/ cheese herb mixture/shredded cheese). Overlap 4 lasagna noodles on top, spread evenly with remaining meat sauce and top with remaining shredded cheese. Sprinkle remaining 1 tablespoon of Italian herb blend evenly over the shredded cheese. Bake for 1 hour or until golden brown on top. Let rest for 15 minutes before serving.

Other Conscious Options:

Take out the meat to make a Starch meal

Cut down half the cheese for less dairy

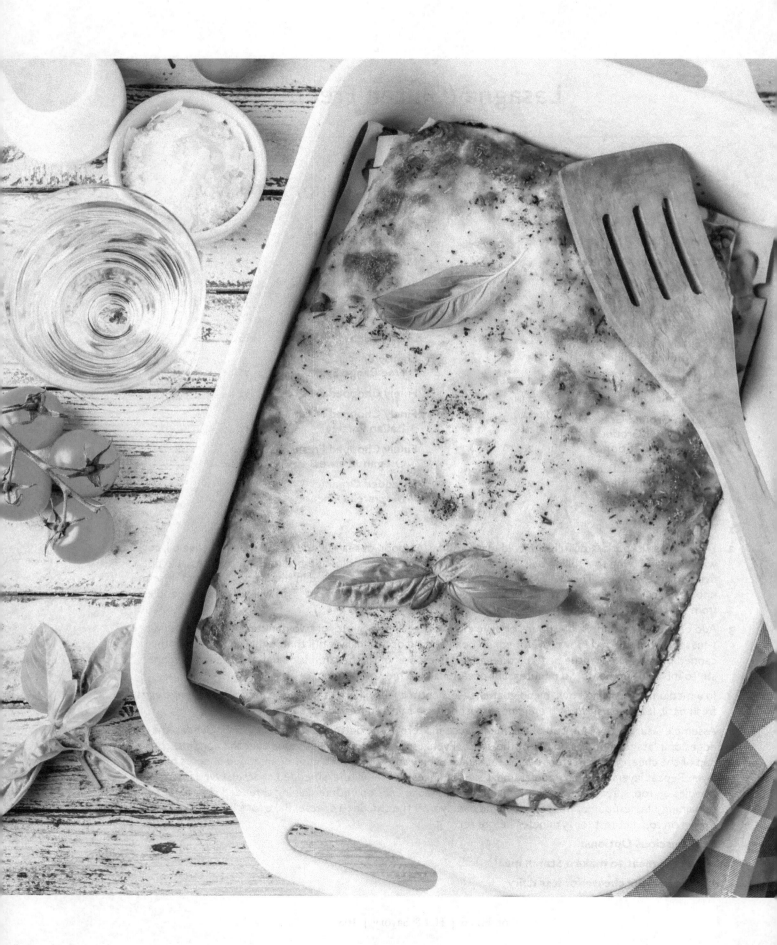

Lox Breakfast

(15 Minutes)

This breakfast is great to implement when you have a busy day and need support.

🔥 SERVED HOT

🍃 SAVORY

INGREDIENTS:

Brown Rice Bread	**2** slices
Coconut Oil	**1** tspn
Organic Free Range Eggs	**2**
Avocado	**½**
Lox	**4** oz

1   Toast brown rice bread in a skillet with coconut oil. Cook organic free-range eggs; sunny side up.

2   Place toast on plate and top with eggs, lox, and top with avocado. Sprinkle with sea salt and pepper. Serves 2 people.

Quinoa & Egg Muffin

(50 Minutes)

INGREDIENTS:

Water	**1** cup
Quinoa	**½** cup
Olive Oil	**2** tbl
Onion Diced	**1**
Fresh Spinach Leaves	**4** cups
Garlic, Minced	**2** cloves
Sea Salt & Fresh Ground Pepper (To Taste)	
Crumbled Feta Cheese, Goat Cheddar Cheese (Optional) — Raw, Goat Cheddar Is Our Recommendation	**1** cup
Flat Leaf Parsley	**¼** cup
Organic Free-Range Eggs, Lightly Beaten	**4** large

A McMuffin Substitute with similar texture.

SERVED HOT

SAVORY

1   Preheat oven to 375° F. Spray a muffin tin with cooking spray and set aside.

2   Combine water and quinoa in a small saucepan and bring to a boil; lower to a simmer, cover, and continue to cook for 15 minutes.

3   In a large frying pan, heat olive oil over medium heat. Add onions and cook until translucent, 3-4 minutes. Stir in spinach leaves and garlic. Season with sea salt and pepper and continue to cook until spinach is wilted; about 2 more minutes. Remove from heat and let cool.

4   In a large mixing bowl, combine cooked quinoa, spinach mixture, cheeses, and parsley. Make sure the quinoa mixture is not warm; if it is, give it a few minutes to cool. Pour in the beaten organic free-range eggs and mix until well combined.

5   Divide batter evenly among prepared muffin cups.

6   Bake for 25 to 30 minutes or until tops are golden brown.

Organic Eggs in a Hole

(10 Minutes)

*Love this breakfast for
kids and
the kid in all of us.*

INGREDIENTS:

Sprouted Grain Bread	**2** slices
Unsalted Butter	**1** tbl
Organic Free Range Eggs	**2** large
Coarse Sea Salt	**1** pinch
Ground Black Pepper (To Taste)	

🔥 SERVED HOT

🌙 SAVORY

1 Spread the bread, both sides, with about half of the butter. Put the rest of the butter into a skillet, large enough to hold both slices of bread side-by-side, and melt it over medium heat.

2 Use a round cookie or biscuit cutter to cut a hole in the center of each slice of buttered bread. Now you have two little buttered "lids!"

3 Cook organic free-range eggs to your liking and serve in the hole of the bread.

Pesto Pizza

(35 Minutes)

INGREDIENTS:

Pine Nuts, Toasted	**2** tbl
Garlic, Finely Chopped (large Clove)	**1**
Kosher Salt	
Chopped Fresh Basil Leaves	**¼** cup
Parmesan	**2** tbl
Extra-Virgin Olive Oil	**2** tbl
Freshly Ground Black Pepper	
Arrowhead Mills Gluten Free Pizza Crust Mix	
Red Onion (Thinly Sliced)	**¼** small
Red Ripe Tomato (Thinly Sliced)	**1**
Kalamata Olives, Pitted And Chopped	**¼** cup
Fresh Mozzarella	**4** slices

Pesto is a great alternative to tomato sauce. Pesto has healthy fat to combine with the starch of the crust.

🔥 SERVED HOT

◐ SAVORY

1 Make the pesto: place the toasted pine nuts in Emulsifying Blender. Add in the garlic and a pinch of kosher salt and combine. Blend in the basil and Parmesan. Stir in the olive oil and season with pepper.

2 Follow directions for pizza crust. Spread the pesto over the dough, leaving 1-inch around the edge to form a crust. Top with the onion and tomato slices and season with kosher salt and pepper. Scatter the olives all over the pizza and top with the fresh mozzarella. Slide the pizza onto the stone and bake until the cheese is melted and the crust is golden, about 8 to 10 minutes.

Rice with Coconut Crusted Salmon
& Coconut Curry Sauce

(50 Minutes)

CILANTRO SCENTED RICE

Chicken Stock	¾ cup
Rice	½ cup
Lime Juice, Fresh	2 tbl
Lime, Zest	1 tspn
Cilantro, Finely Chopped	1 tbl
Sea Salt	½ tspn

COCONUT CRUSTED SALMON

Unsweetened Coconut, Shredded	1¼ cups
Wild Salmon Fillets	4x6 oz
Sea Salt & Pepper (To Taste)	

COCONUT CURRY SAUCE

Coconut Milk	1 cup
Curry Paste	1-2 tbl
Sweet Chile Sauce	1-2 tbl
Bragg's Liquid Amino Acid	2 tbl
Juice Of Lime	1
Organic Raw Honey	1 tspn
Cilantro Finely Chopped	1 bunch

One of my all time favorites!

🔥 SERVED HOT

🌙 SAVORY

Cilantro Scented Rice:

1   Bring water, rice, lime juice, cilantro, and sea salt to a boil in a small saucepan. Reduce heat to low, cover, and cook 20 minutes. Discard cilantro before serving.

Coconut Crusted Salmon:

1   Preheat oven to 375° F. Put coconut into a freezer bag. Drop in the salmon fillets one at a time and toss to coat. Place on a lightly-oiled baking sheet and season with sea salt and pepper. Bake for 15 minutes.

Coconut Curry Sauce:

1   Mix all the ingredients together except for the cilantro. Mix well and heat until it reaches the proper temperature. Pour over the seafood. Garnish with cilantro.

Salmon & Rice Bowl

(38 Minutes)

INGREDIENTS:

Water	**1**	tbl
Broccoli Florets	**2**	cups
Olive Oil	**2**	tspn
Shallot, Minced	**1**	
Bragg's Liquid Amino Acids	**2**	tspn
Grated Fresh Ginger	**1**	tbl
(4-oz) Wild Salmon Fillets, Skinned	**4**	
Brown Rice	**2**	cups
Black Sesame Seeds		

This is a great option to make at home or order out!

🔥 SERVED HOT

🌙 SAVORY

---

1 Heat olive oil in a pan over medium-high heat. Add minced shallot and cook about 1 minute or until golden. Add Bragg's Liquid Aminos and grated fresh ginger; stir.

2 In 2 batches, add salmon fillets and cook for 6 minutes per side or until opaque. Transfer salmon to a plate using a wide spatula; keep warm.

3 Cook brown rice, top with salmon and sprinkle with black sesame seeds; serve.

Stuffed Red Peppers with Rice

(47 Minutes)

You will be very satisfied after this gorgeous meal.

🔥 SERVED HOT

🌙 SAVORY

INGREDIENTS:

Olive Oil	**1** tbl
Oregano, Dried	**1** tspn
Leeks, Chopped	**1⅔** cups
Swiss Chard Leaves, Chopped, Loosely Packed	**6** cups
Sea Salt & Pepper	
Wild Rice, Cooked	**3** cups
Organic Free-Range Eggs, Beaten	**2**
Red Peppers, Sweet	**4**
Feta, Crumbled	**4-6** oz

1. Heat oil in a large, deep skillet over medium heat. Add the oregano, leeks, and cook, stirring occasionally, until leeks are nearly tender.

2. Raise heat to medium-high, add chard and season it generously with sea salt and pepper. Cook, tossing occasionally, until chard is wilted and tender. Let cool, then stir in wild rice and organic free-range eggs. Heat oven to 350° F.

3. Cut the red peppers in half through the stems, so that you end up with 8 pepper "boats" with rounded bottoms. Stuff the pepper halves with the filling, mounding it up slightly in each one. Place stuffed peppers to fit snugly in a baking dish.

4. Spoon a few tablespoons of water into the bottom of dish and cover it tightly with foil.

5. Bake 20-25 minutes, then remove the foil. Sprinkle feta over the peppers and continue to bake, uncovered, another 15-20 minutes. Serve hot, right from the oven.

Thai Food: Spicy Shrimp & Coconut Rice

(28 Minutes)

INGREDIENTS:

Shredded Coconut, Unsweetened	**1** cup
Chicken Stock Or Broth	**2½** cups
Long Grain White Rice	**1** cup
Sea Salt	**1** tspn
Coconut Oil	**2** tbl
Jumbo Shrimp, Peeled & Deveined	**2** lbs
Red Bell Pepper, Seeded & Thinly Sliced	**1**
Fresh Red Chili, Seeded & Thinly Sliced (or ½ teaspoon Red Pepper Flakes)	**1**
Garlic, Finely Chopped	**3** cloves
Fish Sauce (or 2-3 tbl Bragg's Liquid Amino Acid)	**1-1½** tspn
Basil, Torn (A Couple Of Handfuls)	**2** cups
Zest & Juice Of Lime	**1**

Have a night in with easy to make Thai food.

🔥 SERVED HOT

🌑 SAVORY

1. Toast coconut in a saucepan over medium heat until it turns golden brown. Reserve 1/2 cup for garnish.

2. Toss the remaining coconut in the saucepan, add the chicken stock, rice, and sea salt; bring to a boil. Once at a boil, reduce the heat to a simmer, place a lid on top, and cook for 15 minutes. Let the mixture stand for 5 minutes off the heat then fluff with a fork.

3. While the rice is cooking, preheat a large, nonstick skillet over high heat with coconut oil. When the pan is hot, add the shrimp, red bell peppers, chili (or red pepper flakes), and garlic, stirring frequently for about 3-4 minutes.

4. Add the fish sauce (or Bragg's Liquid Amino) and toss with basil to combine. Serve the shrimp and some of the sauce over the coconut rice and squeeze some lime juice over everything. Garnish with the reserved toasted coconut and lime zest.

Vegetarian Tacos

(18 Minutes)

A great vegetarian option for taco cravings.

🔥 SERVED HOT

🌙 SAVORY

INGREDIENTS:

Coconut Oil	**2** tbl
Butternut Squash	**1**
Ground Cumin	**½** tspn
Kosher Salt & Black Pepper	
(16-oz) Can Of Black Beans, Soaked & Rinsed	**1**
Organic Corn Tortillas, Warmed	**8**
Red Onions	**1–2** small
Goat Cheese	**1** cup
Parsley	**¼** cup
Lime Wedges	

1   Heat the oil in a large skillet over medium heat. Add the squash, cumin, 1/2 teaspoon kosher salt, and 1/4 teaspoon pepper and cook, stirring occasionally, until tender; 11-13 minutes. Add the beans and 1/4 cup water and cook until heated through; 1-2 minutes.

2   Top the tortillas with the squash, beans, onion, cheese, and parsley, dividing evenly. Serve with lime wedges (if desired).

Vegan Buddha Bowl

(30 Minutes)

INGREDIENTS:

Cumin Seed, Ground	1 tspn
Quinoa, Rinsed	1 cup
Salt, Divided	1¾ tspn
Sweet Potatoes, Scrubbed & Chopped (No Need To Peel)	2 large
(15½-oz) Chickpeas, Rinsed & Drained	1 can
Olive Oil	1 tbl
Salt	¾ tspn
Lacinato Kale, Stems Removed, Chopped (About 10 Large Leaves)	1 bunch
Lime, Juiced	1
Garlic, Minced	1 clove
Ripe Avocados	2
Roasted Pumpkin Seeds	½ cup

A bowl that will help you feel full and satiated.

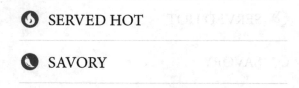

 SERVED HOT

 SAVORY

1 In a medium pot, combine quinoa, 1/4 teaspoon salt, and 2 cups water. Bring to a boil over high heat, then reduce to a low simmer. Cook quinoa for about 10 minutes, until water is absorbed and quinoa is fluffy. Fluff quinoa with a fork.

2 Preheat oven to 425° F. On a sheet pan, toss sweet potatoes and chickpeas with olive oil, cumin, and 3/4 teaspoon salt. Bake for 25-30 minutes, until chickpeas are crispy and sweet potatoes are soft.

3 In a medium bowl, sprinkle kale evenly with remaining 3/4 teaspoon salt. Massage salt into kale for 15 seconds to break down the tough leaves. Add lime juice and garlic, tossing to combine.

4 In a separate medium bowl, mash avocados. Add guacamole mix sauce to the avocados, and stir to combine.

5 To each single serving bowl, add a base layer of quinoa, kale, sweet potato, and chickpeas then top with guacamole and pumpkin seeds.

Heather's Healthy French Toast

(10 Minutes)

When you have a Combined Meal
for breakfast, try having the other
Meal Types for the rest of the day.

🔥 SERVED HOT

🍓 SWEET

INGREDIENTS:

Sprouted Grain Bread	2 slices
Whole Organic Free Range Eggs	2
Almond Milk	⅛ cup
Cinnamon	to taste
Organic Vanilla Extract	½ tspn
Maple Syrup	2 tbl
Coconut Oil	1 tspn
Ghee	to taste

1 Mix organic free-range eggs, almond milk, cinnamon, and vanilla extract in a bowl. Dip the bread until thoroughly moist.

2 Toast bread in a heated skillet with coconut oil until golden brown on each side.

3 Top with organic butter, ghee, or almond butter and organic maple syrup.

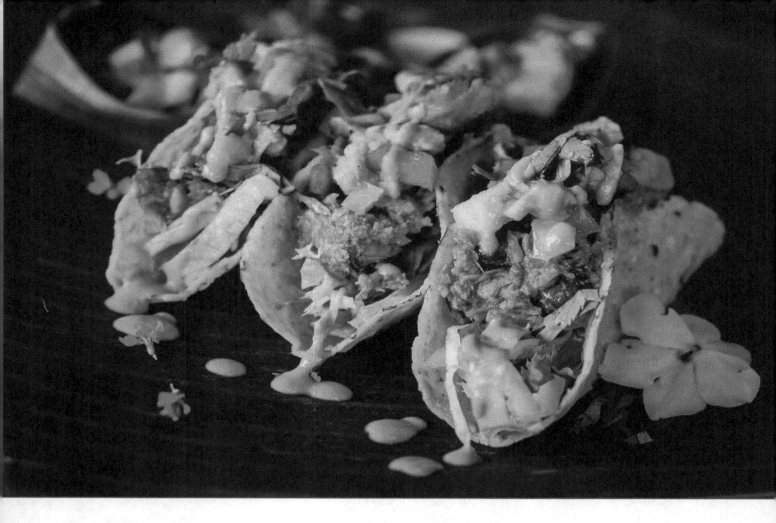

🌱 Vegan Meals

These meals include vegetables and healthy fats and do not follow either side of the tree. Compliment them with Main Meals or use as an appetizer. These meals may still contribute to your total daily exchanges.

Total Daily Exchanges is part of the Conscious Nutrition Program to support you with how much to eat of the Food Groups from the Conscious Nutrition Food Tree.

Enjoy!

Artichoke Soup

(30 Minutes)

This recipe is the new vegan version of chicken noodle soup. I am in love with it and it feels so nourishing and hydrating.

🔥 SERVED HOT

🌑 SAVORY

INGREDIENTS:

Artichoke Halves	**3** cans
Carrots	**4** large
Celery	**1** bunch
Veggie Broth	**32** oz
Salt & Pepper (To Taste)	

1 Sauté carrots and celery in coconut oil for 5 minutes. Add artichoke heart, seasonings, and broth and simmer for 30 minutes. Enjoy!

Carrot/Coconut & Lime Soup

(40 Minutes)

INGREDIENTS:

Carrots, Peeled & Roughly Chopped	½ lb
Onion, Peeled & Roughly Chopped	1
Coconut Oil	1 tbl
Veggie Stock	2 cups
Coconut Milk	4 cups
Lime Zest	1 lime
Lime Juice	½ lime
Turmeric	¼ tspn
Cayenne	¼ tspn
Salt & Pepper (To Taste)	

Put the lime in the coconut and enjoy!

SERVED HOT

SAVORY

1   Heat coconut oil in a Dutch oven or large soup pot.

2   Once hot, add onions and carrots and let sweat for approximately 10-15 minutes until the carrots start to soften and the onion is translucent.

3   Add the stock, turmeric, cayenne, and lime zest and bring to a boil; allow the pot to simmer for approximately 20 minutes.

4   Once the carrots are soft, turn off the heat and add the coconut milk. Use an immersion blender or add to your blender and blend until smooth.

5   Gently reheat the soup for about 5-10 minutes. Add the lime juice and season with salt and pepper to taste.

Carrot Ginger Soup

(40 Minutes)

*When I first made this
homemade, I loved it and now
is a winter staple.*

SERVED HOT

SAVORY

INGREDIENTS:

Coconut Oil	**1** tbl
Yellow Onion, Chopped	**1** medium
Garlic Minced	**1** clove
Fresh Ginger, Chopped	**3** tbl
Carrots, Peeled & Chopped (Baby Carrots Are Also Fine)	**1** lb
Vegetable Stock	**32** oz
(14-oz) Coconut Cream Or Coconut Milk	**1** can
Salt (To Taste)	**½** tspn

1   Begin by heating up a large skillet to medium-high heat. Melt the coconut oil.

2   Add onion, garlic, and ginger. Cook until fragrant and onion is almost clear; about 5 minutes.

3   Add carrots and vegetable stock; bring to a boil.

4   Reduce heat to simmer. Cook until carrots are nice and soft, about 25 minutes. Slowly stir in coconut milk or coconut cream.

5   With an immersion blender, blend soup until smooth. You can also use a regular blender and blend in batches. Add salt to taste. Serve hot!

Cauliflower & Spinach Casserole

(30 Minutes)

INGREDIENTS:

Cauliflower Florets, About 1 Third Of A Small Head	**6** oz
Cashew Milk	**6** oz
Coconut Oil	**2** tbl
Onion, Finely Chopped	**1** medium
Garlic, Minced	**3** cloves
Freshly Grated Nutmeg	**½** tspn
Spinach, Washed Well & Roughly Chopped	**1** lb
Kosher Salt & Freshly Ground Black Pepper	

Clears while supporting blood sugar balancing.
This casserole is one of my favorites to have when you need cozy and comforting.

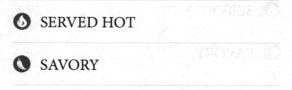 SERVED HOT

SAVORY

1   Combine cauliflower and milk in a small saucepan. Bring to a simmer over medium heat, cover, reduce heat to lowest setting, and let cook until cauliflower is completely tender, about 10 minutes. Blend into a smooth purée using an immersion blender or countertop blender. Set aside.

2   Heat coconut oil over medium heat in a large saucepan until melted. Add onion and cook, stirring frequently, until softened but not browned, about 4 minutes. Add garlic and cook, stirring constantly, until fragrant, about 30 seconds. Add nutmeg and stir to combine. Add spinach one handful at a time, stirring and folding until each handful of spinach is wilted before adding the next.

3   Add cauliflower purée to spinach mixture and stir to combine. Bring to a bare simmer and cook, stirring occasionally, until spinach is completely tender and mixture is creamy. Season to taste with salt and pepper and serve.

Dairy-Free Cream of Asparagus Soup

(19 Minutes)

Asparagus and soups are great for your soul.

🔥 SERVED HOT

🌿 SAVORY

INGREDIENTS:

Asparagus Trimmed Into 2 Inch Pieces With A Dozen Tips Reserved For Garnish	**2** lbs
Cauliflower, Cored & Chopped	**½** head
Onion, Diced	**1**
Garlic, Minced	**3** cloves
Ghee	**4** tbl
Olive Oil	**1** tbl
Chicken Stock	**4** cups
Lemon, Quartered	**1**
Sea Salt & Black Pepper (To Taste)	

1 Bring a Dutch oven to medium-high heat. Melt the ghee and add the onion. Sauté until the onion is translucent, about 7-8 minutes.

2 Add the garlic and cook until fragrant; about 30 seconds.

3 Add the chopped asparagus and a large pinch of salt and pepper. Sauté until the asparagus is slightly tender; 5-6 minutes.

4 Boil 1/2 head of cauliflower until tender in chicken stock.

5 Discard/ drain chicken stock. Keep 1 cup for liquid if needed for desired consistency.

6 Blend all of the ingredients together.

7 Top with Ghee and squeeze the lemon.

8 Enjoy!

Mushroom & Chestnut Burgers

(80 Minutes)

INGREDIENTS:

Black Beans, Canned, Mashed	1⅓ cups
Olive Oil (Plus Extra For Frying)	1 tbl
Mushrooms, Cremini/White Button, Finely Chopped	6–8 medium
Celery, Finely Chopped	1 stalk
Carrot, Finely Chopped	1 small
Red Onion, Finely Chopped	¼ onion
Garlic, Finely Minced	2 cloves
Salt	½ tspn
Chia Seeds, Ground	1 tbl
Bragg's Soy Sauce	2½ tbl
Nutritional Yeast	2 tbl
Lemon Juice	1 squeeze
Optional Gluten Free Bread Crumbs Or Flour	

This burgers satisfies your savory and umami taste buds and cravings from the Conscious Nutrition Cravings Book.

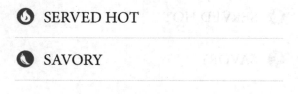 SERVED HOT

SAVORY

1 In a large skillet, heat olive oil over medium-high heat and sauté the finely chopped mushrooms, celery, carrot, onion, and garlic until just tender. Sprinkle with salt and stir.

2 Add the black beans, ground chia seeds, nutritional yeast, and soy sauce, lemon juice and stir until the mixture gets very thick and difficult to mix. You can add in gluten-free bread crumbs or flour here if your mixture doesn't get thick enough. Refrigerate for at least 1 hour.

3 Take the mixture and make patties.

4 Fry in olive oil until golden brown on both sides.

5 Place on salad or bun, top with your favorite toppings and enjoy

Organic Vegetable Soup

(15 Minutes)

This is a great soup to prepare on weekends to have ready during the week as a quick appetizer or with meals.

🔥 SERVED HOT

🌙 SAVORY

INGREDIENTS:

Vegetable Broth, Organic	**1** qt
Diced Vegetables	**4** cups
Yellow Onion	**½**
Carrot	**1** medium
Kale Leaves	**1** handful
Zucchini	**1** medium
Tomato	**1** medium
Spinach	**1** handful
Green Beans	**1** handful
Chopped Fresh Herbs (Basil & Italian Parsley)	**2** tbl
Freshly Ground Black Pepper & Sea Salt (To Taste)	

1 In a medium soup pot, heat broth to a boil, then reduce to simmer.

2 Add onion, carrots, and simmer covered for 2 minutes. Add remaining vegetables and simmer until just tender.

3 Add fresh herbs, sea salt, and pepper to taste.

Roasted Brussels Sprouts & Mushrooms

(40 Minutes)

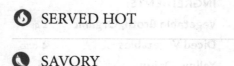

🔥 SERVED HOT

☯ SAVORY

This meal can be a side dish or when you are hungry but do not need a protein or starch.

INGREDIENTS:

Brussels Sprouts, Trimmed & Halved Lengthwise	**3** lb
Olive Oil	¼ cup
Maple Syrup, Grade B	½ cup
Minced Garlic	½ tbl
Sea Salt	
Cracked Pepper	
Olive Oil	**1** cup
Large Shallots (About 6),	½ lb
Cut Crosswise Into 1/8 Inch Thick Slices Separated Intro Rings (2 ½ Cups)	

FOR MUSHROOMS:

Unsalted Butter Or Coconut Oil	¾ stick (6 tbl)
Shiitake Mushrooms Or Mixed Fresh Wild Mushrooms Such As Chanterelle & Oyster, Trimmed, Quartered If Large	1¼ lb
Dry White Wine	¼ cup
Chopped Fresh Thyme	1 tbl
Chopped Fresh Marjoram	1 tbl
Salt	½ tspn
Black Pepper	¼ tspn
Water	½ cup

1 Put oven rack in upper third of oven and preheat oven to 450 F.

2 Line 2 shallow baking sheet with tin foil, and place in oven.

3 Toss Brussels sprouts with olive oil, maple syrup, garlic salt, and pepper.

4 Roast, stirring occasionally and switching position of pans halfway through roasting, until tender, browned, and a little crispy about, 25 to 35 minutes.

Fry Shallots while Brussels Sprouts Roast:

5 Heat oil in a 10-inch heavy skillet over moderate heat until temperature reaches then fry shallots in 3 batches, until golden brown, 3 to 5 minutes per batch

6 Quickly transfer with a slotted spoon to paper towels to drain, spreading in a single layer. Pour off oil from skillet.

Sauté Mushrooms and Assemble Dish:

1 Heat 5 tablespoons butter in skillet over moderately high heat until foam subsides, then sauté mushrooms, stirring occasionally, until golden brown and tender, about 7 minutes.

2 Add wine, thyme, marjoram, salt, and pepper and simmer, uncovered, stirring occasionally, until liquid is reduced to a glaze, about 2 minutes.

3 Add water (1/2 cup) and remaining tablespoon butter and simmer, swirling skillet, until butter is melted.

4 Transfer to a serving dish and stir in Brussels sprouts. Sprinkle with some of shallots and serve with remaining shallots on the side.

Roasted Veggies

(40 Minutes)

This is something you can do every week when you have extra veggies to bake and use as a side dish.

⬤ SERVED HOT

⬤ SAVORY

INGREDIENTS:

Brussels Sprouts, Sliced In Half	1 cup
Beets, Chunked	3
Onion, Chunked	1 large
Leek, Sliced	1
Broccoli Head	½
Bell Pepper (Any Color But Green)	1
Cauliflower, Chunked	¼
Avocado Oil	2 tbl
Sea Salt & Pepper	

1 Place veggies on a cookie sheet.

2 Drizzle oil, salt, and pepper.

3 Bake for 30-40 minutes at 350° F.

Spring Veggie Stew

(25 Minutes)

Keep this stew recipe handy to cook all of the veggies in your crisper.

🔥 SERVED HOT

🌿 SAVORY

INGREDIENTS:

Asparagus, White Cut Into Thin, 1-Inch Lengths	¼ lb
Cranberry Beans, Shelled Fresh (4-oz Or 1 lb In The Pod)	1 cup
Olive Oil , Extra-Virgin	2 tbl
Scallions, Thin White & Pale Green Parts Only	20
Mushrooms, Beech (Available At Asian Or Specialty Food Markets)	¼ lb
Sea Salt	
Turnips, White About 2 Inches In Diameter, Peeled & Cut Into Wedges	6
Carrots Cut Into 1-Inch-Long Sticks	2 medium
Vegetable Stock	2¼ cups
Zucchini Halved Lengthwise & Sliced Crosswise 1/4 Inch Thick	6 oz
Finely Grated Lemon Zest	½ tspn
Fresh Lemon Juice	1 tspn
Romaine Heart Cut Into 2-Inch Pieces	1
Minced Chives	1 tbl

1 In a medium pot of simmering salted water, cook the asparagus over moderately high heat until tender; about 4 minutes. Using a slotted spoon, transfer the asparagus to a bowl. Add the cranberry beans to the water and simmer over moderate heat until tender; about 40 minutes. Drain the beans and transfer to the bowl.

2 Meanwhile, in a medium-enameled, cast-iron casserole, heat 1/2 tablespoon of olive oil. Add the scallions and cook over moderate heat until barely tender; about 1 minute. Transfer the scallions to the bowl with asparagus. Add another 1/2 tablespoon of olive oil to the casserole. Add the mushrooms, season with salt, cover, and cook over moderate heat, stirring a few times, until lightly browned and tender; about 3 minutes. Transfer the mushrooms to the bowl.

3 Heat the remaining 1 tablespoon of olive oil in the casserole. Add the turnips and carrots, season with salt and cook over moderate heat for 1 minute. Add 1 cup of stock, cover, and cook over low heat, stirring occasionally, for 15 minutes. Add another 1/2 cup stock, cover, and cook until the turnips and carrots are tender; about 10 minutes longer. Add the zucchini, 1/2 cup stock, and simmer until the zucchini is just tender; about 4 minutes. Add the remaining 1/4 cup stock to the casserole along with the lemon zest, lemon juice, and lettuce and cook, stirring, until the lettuce just wilts; about 20 seconds.

4 Add the asparagus, beans, scallions, and mushrooms to the stew. Simmer briefly, until heated through; about 30 seconds. Add the chives and serve the stew in bowls.

Spaghetti Squash with Pesto

(25 Minutes)

One of my favorite meals or side dishes.

SERVED HOT

SAVORY

INGREDIENTS:

Spaghetti Squash	1
Halved Lengthwise & Seeded	
Onion, Sliced	1
Kale	1 cup
Stems Removed & Leaves Chopped	
White Mushrooms, Sliced	4
Italian Seasoning	1 tspn
Red Pepper Flakes	1 tspn
Olive Oil	1 tspn
Dairy Free Pesto	2 tbl
(Make Your Own Pesto In Emulsifying Blender)	

1 Preheat oven to 400° F. Grease a baking sheet.

2 Place squash, skin side down on prepared baking sheet. Bake until cooked through, about 1 hour. Remove from oven; cool for 10 minutes. Once squash is cool enough to handle, scrape flesh into string-like strands with a fork. Place in a bowl and set aside.

3 Melt 1 tablespoon of olive oil in a large skillet over medium-high heat. Add onion; cook and stir until onion begins to turn translucent. Stir in kale and mushrooms; reduce heat to medium-low.

4 Stir in squash, remaining 2 tablespoons butter, garlic salt, Italian seasoning, and red pepper flakes; cook for 2 minutes. Remove from stove and place squash mixture in a large bowl.

5 Make your own Pesto (recipe on page 160) in emulsifying blender and stir olive oil and pesto into the squash mixture.

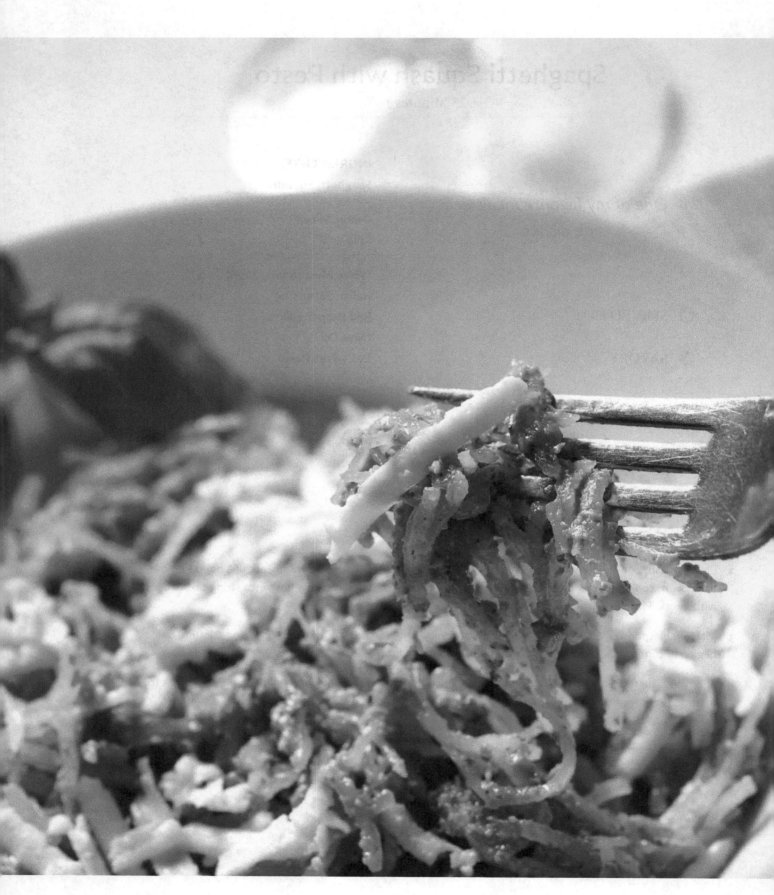

Tomato Basil Soup with Zucchini

(17 Minutes)

We all grew up on tomato soup and grilled cheese sandwiches. This soup will support those memories.

🔥 SERVED HOT

🌑 SAVORY

INGREDIENTS:

Olive Oil	**2** tbl
Leeks, Sliced	**2**
Carrots Diced Coarse	**2** medium
Celery, Stalk Diced Coarse	**1** medium
Garlic, Minced	**2** cloves
Tomatoes Peeled, Seeded, & Chopped Coarse	**4** large
Sea Salt & Pepper (To Taste)	
Zucchini Cut Into 1/4-Inch Dice	**2** medium
Basil Leaf (Fresh), Shredded	**¼** cup
Vegetable Broth	**32** oz

1   Heat oil in a large soup kettle. Add onions, carrots, and celery. Sauté until vegetables soften; about 5 minutes. Add garlic and sauté until fragrant; about 1 minute. Add broth and simmer for about 1-2 minutes.

2   With the soup base at a simmer, add tomatoes, sea salt to taste, and simmer for 30 minutes. Add zucchini and simmer for 10 minutes. Pulse in emulsifying blender until desired consistency is reached (if you are looking for a more rustic soup no need to blend). Stir in shredded basil. Season with additional sea salt if necessary and pepper to taste.

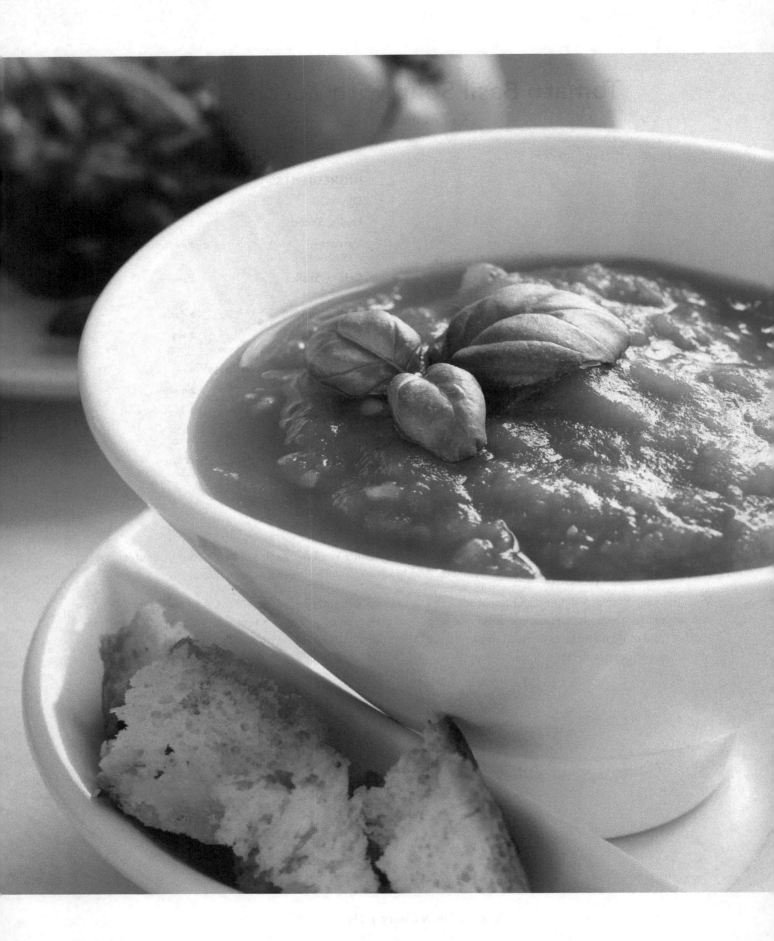

Chunky Tomato Soup

(20 Minutes)

This soup satisfies all of your taste buds and cravings from the Conscious Nutrition Cravings Book, such as creamy and savory.

🔥 SERVED HOT

⚫ SAVORY

INGREDIENTS:

Coconut Oil	1 tbl
Onion, Chopped	1
Garlic, Crushed	1 tspn
Oregano	1 tspn
Basil, Dried	1 tspn
(14-oz) Cans Whole Peeled Tomatoes	2 cans
Coconut Sugar	2 tbl
Vegetable Stock	2 cups
Basil, Fresh (For Serving)	

1 Add the chopped onion and crushed garlic to a pot with coconut oil and sauté. Add in the oregano and dried basil and sauté until the onions are softened.

2 Add the whole peeled tomatoes, sugar, and 2 cups of vegetable stock.

3 Bring to boil and then reduce heat to simmer until all the ingredients are soft and cooked; around 30 minutes.

4 Serve with a sprinkle of dried basil, dried oregano, and fresh basil leaves.

Gilicious Apple Bake

(50 Minutes)

INGREDIENTS:

Chopped Apples *Of Any Variety*	**6** cups
Coconut Milk	**1** can
Garbanzo Bean Flour	**½** cup
Baking Soda	**1** tspn
Cinnamon	**2** tspn

This recipe is inspired by one of my retreaters! This dessert is for special occasions. When you need a pick me up, have friends over and want to indulge. Add some coconut whip cream on top and enjoy.

🔥 SERVED HOT

🍓 SWEET

1   Place apples in an 8x10 pan.

2   Sprinkle the flour, cinnamon, and baking soda on top.

3   Pour the coconut milk over mixture.

4   Bake at 350° F for 45 minutes.

5   Add coconut whip cream on top!

Blended Vegetables

(5 Minutes)

One of my favorites. This will grow on you, and you may actually crave this. It took me awhile to figure out the consistency of this recipe, if you want it thinner, add more ice or water.

INGREDIENTS:

Carrot	1
Celery Stalk	1
Spinach Or Kale	1 cup
Myers Lemon	½
Ginger Root	1 chunk
Water	2 cups

❄ SERVED COLD

◖ SAVORY

1 Cut up vegetables, add water, and blend in an emulsifying blender.

2 This is my favorite way to begin my day!

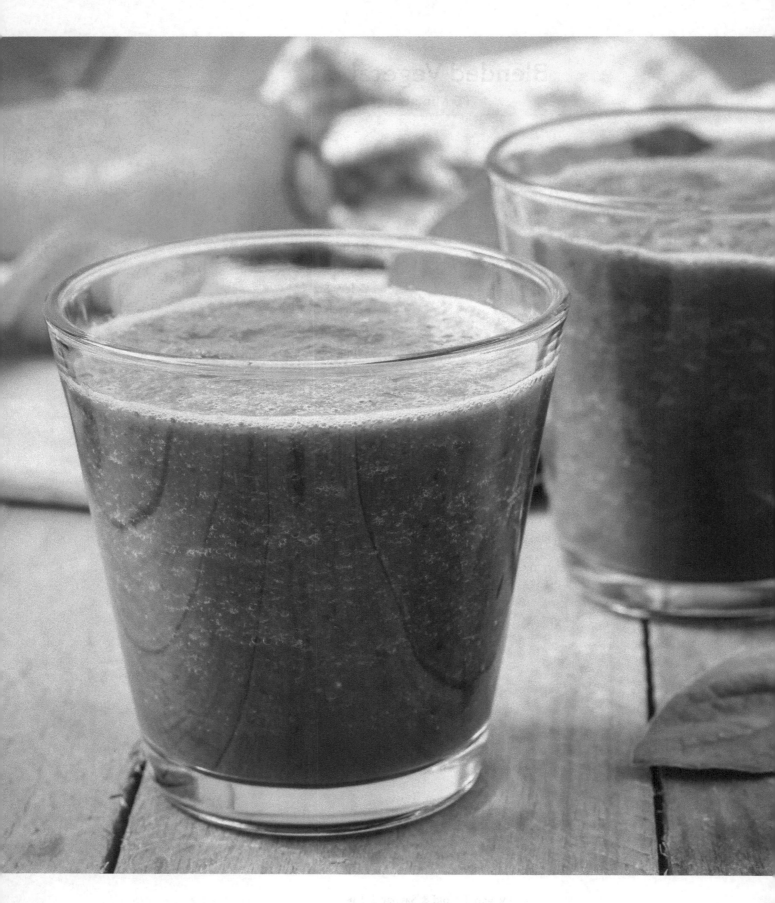

Coconut Wraps

(5 Minutes)

This wrap is inspired by one of my favorite Plant-Based restaurants, Peace Pie in San Diego.

❄ SERVED COLD

🌙 SAVORY

INGREDIENTS:

Coconut Wrap	
Spinach	**1** handful
Hope Hummus **(Coconut Curry)**	**2** tbl
Cucumber **Thinly Sliced Lengthwise**	¼
Mango, Sliced	½
Carrots, Shaved	**3** tbl
Avocado	¼

1 Place wrap on a plate.

2 Smear hummus on half of the wrap.

3 Place cucumbers, mango, avocado, and carrots in a row.

4 Wrap and enjoy!

Coleslaw

(12 Minutes)

INGREDIENTS:

Cabbage, Green	½ head
Cabbage, Red	½ head
Red Onion, **Sliced Thin**	½ small
Pink Lady Apple, **Cored & Sliced Thin**	1
Red Wine Vinegar	1 tbl
Sea Salt	
Fresh Ground Pepper	
Homemade Mayonnaise (See Page 161 For Mayonnaise Recipe)	¼ cup
Cranberries, Dried Organic	¼ cup

Another perfect side dish with grilled meats or on top of salads.

❄ SERVED COLD

◐ SAVORY

1 Remove tough outer leaves and core from cabbage and slice into thin shreds. Place shredded cabbage, sliced onions and apple into a medium-size bowl. In a separate small bowl, whisk together ingredients for dressing.

2 Taste for acid and add sea salt and pepper to taste. Pour dressing over cabbage, apples, onions and toss until completely combined. Stir in cranberries. Taste again for sea salt and pepper. Serve immediately, or chill to allow the flavors to permeate and cabbage to soften.

Fava Bean Pesto

(10 Minutes)

*I LOVE pesto of all sorts. So great
to use as a
dip or topping.*

❄ SERVED COLD

🌙 SAVORY

INGREDIENTS:

Fresh Fava Beans, Shelled	**1** lb
Basil	**1** handful
Parsley	**1** handful
Garlic Clove, Sliced	**1** large
Lemon, Juiced	**½**
Olive Oil	**½** cup
Hemp Seed Hearts	**2** tbl
Salt	
Pepper	

1 First, shell the fresh fava beans out of the pod.

2 Measure out olive oil, and hemp seed hearts.

3 Add fava beans, basil, parsley, hemp seeds hearts, garlic, grated cheese, and juice of 1/2 lemon to a blender or food processor. Begin to blend at medium speed.

4 At the opening of the blender or food processor, slowly stream in olive oil adding more, or less, depending on the consistency of preference.

5 Once ingredients achieve pesto consistency, stop blending and add a pinch of salt and pepper to taste. Blend all ingredients one final time to incorporate spices.

6 Grab your favorite crunchy veggies to dip.

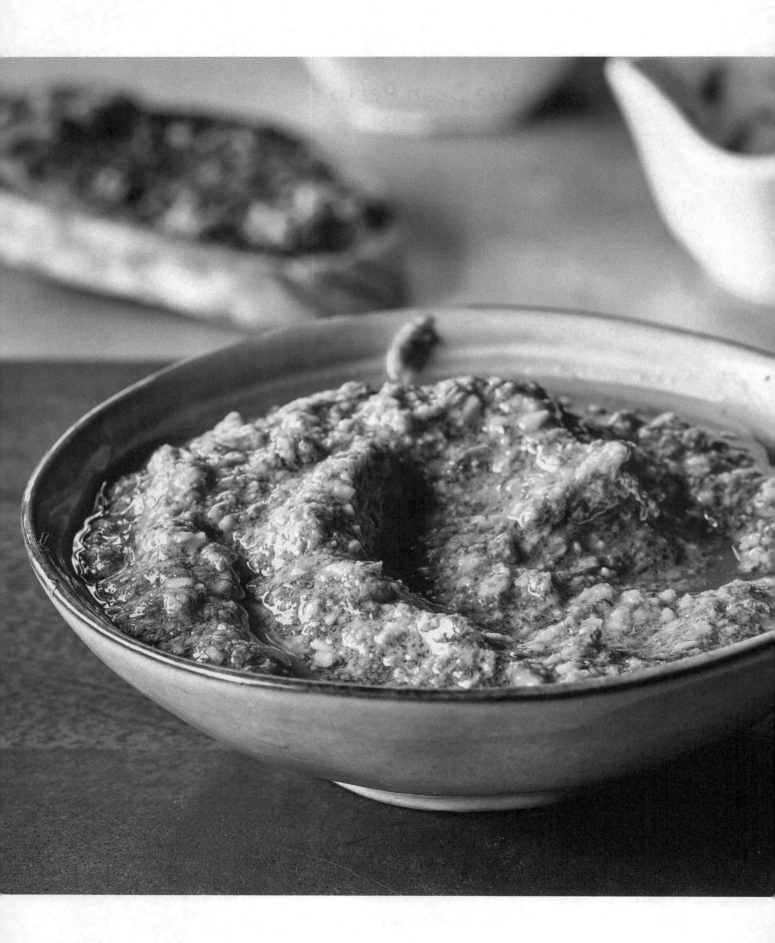

Kohrabi Side Dish

(35 Minutes)

I was so curious about this vegetable, I had to try it. It tastes like a radish and turnip combined.

❄ SERVED COLD

◗ SAVORY

THE DRESSING:

Evoo Olive Oil	**3** tbl
Cider Vinegar	**3** tbl
Garlic Clove	**1** large
Cumin Seeds, Whole	**1** tspn
Lemon- Juice Only	**1** large
Ground Black Pepper (To Taste)	

THE SALAD:

Kohlrabi Or Two Smaller Ones	**1** large
Radishes	**10–12**
Carrots	**4**
Seed Mix — Pumpkin & Sunflower Seeds Are A Great Choice	**1** handful

1 Mix all of the ingredients for the dressing in a large bowl and put to one side. Peel the Kohlrabi, then thinly slice it using a sharp knife. Place the slices of Kohlrabi into the bowl of dressing and mix to coat.

2 Wash and peel the carrots and radishes, then thinly slice them, add Kohlrabi and leave this in the bowl for approximately 30 minutes. Then add a sprinkle of seeds to garnish.

3 Finally, drizzle the dressing from the bowl over the platter and then serve.

Pickled Broccoli Stems

(12 Minutes)

INGREDIENTS:

Broccoli Stems (From One Bunch)	**3**
Garlic, Peeled & Smashed	**1** clove
Black Peppercorns	**½** tspn

BASIC BRINE:

White Vinegar	**1** cup
Water	**1** cup
Kosher Salt	**1** tbl
Sugar	**2** tbl
Organic Coconut	

I always keep the broccoli stems to dip in hummus and am now doing this!

❄ SERVED COLD

🌙 SAVORY

1   Peel the broccoli stems and cut, either crosswise into rounds, or lengthwise into stalks. Pack the stems tightly in a mason jar, along with the garlic clove and the black peppercorns, making sure to leave 1/2-inch of headspace.

2   In a small, non-reactive saucepan, heat the vinegar, water, salt, and sugar, stirring until the sugar and salt are dissolved. Remove from heat and let the brine cool for about 5 minutes.

3   Fill each jar to within 1/2-inch of the top of the jar with brine. This recipe makes enough brine for 1 quart.

4   Let the jars cool to room temperature. Store the pickles in the fridge. They will taste good after 24 hours, but are best after at least 2 days. They will keep up to one month.

Ribboned Carrot Salad with Spice

(12 Minutes)

When you crave more spice, flavor, and freshness with or for your meal.

❄ SERVED COLD

🌙 SAVORY

INGREDIENTS:

Black Sesame Seeds	**1** tspn
Garlic Powder	**½** tspn
Cumin Seed	**¼** tspn
Coriander Seed	**¼** tspn
Paprika	**½** tspn
Pistachios, Raw Shelled	**¾** cup
Carrots, Peeled (About 1 Pound)	**8** large
Parsley, Fresh, Finely Chopped, Plus More For Topping	**½** cup
Olive Oil, Extra Virgin	**4** tbl
Sherry Vinegar	**3** tbl
Lemon Juice, Fresh	**1** tbl
Kosher Salt	**¼** tspn

1　Preheat oven to 350° F.

2　On a small, rimmed baking sheet, spread pistachios evenly and toast for 5-7 minutes, or until fragrant. Set aside to cool.

To Make The Dressing:

1　In a small bowl, whisk together olive oil, sherry vinegar, lemon juice, garlic powder, cumin, coriander, paprika and salt, and set aside.

To Make The Salad:

1　Using a vegetable peeler, shave carrots into thin ribbons.

2　In a large salad bowl, combine carrot ribbons, toasted pistachios, and parsley and toss with dressing.

3　Serve with more parsley and feta (optional).

Sweet Pea & Dill Salad

(10 Minutes)

INGREDIENTS:

Green Peas, Blanched	**4** cups
Mayonnaise Or Vegenaise	**½** cup
Prepared Horseradish	**2** tbl
Dijon-Style Prepared Mustard	**1** tbl
Dill Weed, Fresh, Chopped	**¼** cup
Ground Black Pepper (To Taste)	

A great light meal or a side dish. This reminds me of growing up and my mom's lettuce & pea salad that I like.

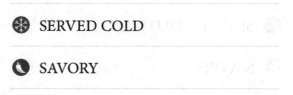 SERVED COLD

SAVORY

1 Gently pat peas with a paper towel to absorb any excess moisture. Place peas in a large bowl.

2 In a small bowl, combine the mayonnaise, horseradish, mustard, and 3 tablespoons dill weed.

3 Add to peas and toss to coat. Sprinkle remaining dill over top.

4 Cover and chill for at least 2 hours before serving.

Thai Spring Rolls

(10 Minutes)

Super fresh and crunchy.
Rice wrappers are minimal starch.

❄ SERVED COLD

🌙 SAVORY

INGREDIENTS:

Small, Round Rice Wrappers (Dried)	1 package
Vermicelli Rice Noodles, Thin Cooked & Run Through With Cold Water, Drained	1–1½ cups
Bean Sprouts	1–2 cups
Thai Basil Or Sweet Basil, Fresh Roughly Chopped	½ cup
Coriander, Fresh Roughly Chopped	½ cup
Carrot, Shredded	¼ cup
Spring Onions Cut Into Matchstick Pieces	3–4
Braggs Liquid Aminos	2 tbl
Rice Vinegar	1 tbl
Fish Sauce (Available At Asian Foods Stores) Or Another Tablespoon Bragg's If Vegetarian	1 tbl
Coconut Palm Sugar	1 tspn

1. Set rice wrappers aside. In a cup, stir together the soy sauce, vinegar, fish sauce (if using), and sugar. Place all other ingredients for the fresh rolls in a large mixing bowl and drizzle the soy sauce mixture over. Toss to mix. Fill a large bowl with hot water (but not boiling, as you'll be dipping your fingers into it). Start by submerging one wrapper into the water. It should soften after 30 seconds.

2. Remove the wrapper and place on a clean surface. Add another wrapper to the hot water as you fill and roll the first one.

3. Place a heaping tablespoon of roll ingredients toward the bottom of the wrapper. Spread the ingredients out horizontally (in the shape of a fresh roll).

4. Fold the sides of the wrapper over the ingredients, bring up the bottom. Tuck the bottom around the ingredients and roll to the top of the wrapper. To secure the roll, wet it with a little water on your fingers and press (like sealing an envelope).

5. To serve, place your platter or bowl of rolls on the table along with the dipping sauce. Eat with your fingers and many napkins. Enjoy!

Vegan Caesar Salad

(5 Minutes)

INGREDIENTS:

Romaine Lettuce	1 head
Hearts Of Palm	1 can
Garlic	1 clove
Dijon Mustard	1 tbl
Capers	1 tbl
Lemon Juice	¼ cup
Salt & Pepper	
Water	¾ cup
Extra Virgin Olive Oil	2 tbl

This crunchy salad is a great side dish or an easy lunch.

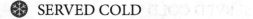

❄ SERVED COLD

🍓 SWEET

1 Chop lettuce.

2 Drain and rinse the hearts of palm and toss with one cup with lettuce.

3 Take the rest of the hearts of palm, garlic, mustard, capers, lemon juice, salt, and pepper and blend to dress the salad.

Vegan Lettuce Wraps

(15 Minutes)

A spectacular appetizer or a light snack in the middle of the day.

❄ SERVED COLD

🍓 SWEET

INGREDIENTS:

Ginger, Chopped	2 tbl
Sesame Or Olive Oil	1 tbl
Celery, Diced	¾ cup
Carrots, Diced	¾ cup
Tamari Or Soy Sauce	2 tbl
Crushed Red Pepper Flakes	½ tspn
Sea Salt & Pepper (To Taste)	
Bibb, Romaine Lettuce, Or Napa Cabbage	1 head
Sesame Seeds	2 tbl

1. Heat oil in sauté pan and add ginger, celery, and carrots. Stir and sauté for 5-7 minutes until slightly soft. Add soy sauce, seasoning, and stir, cooking for 10 minutes.

2. Remove from heat, spoon into lettuce leaves, sprinkle sesame seeds on top, roll and enjoy.

Make A Spicy Peanut Dipping Sauce By Mixing:

1 clove Garlic, Minced
3 tbl Rice Vinegar
1/2 cup Tamari
1-2 tbl Sriracha Or Chili Sauce
1/2 cup Organic Peanut Butter Or Almond Butter
Juice Of One Lime
2 tbl Sesame Oil

Chia Seed Pudding

(5 Minutes to mix. Cool for 3 hours.)

INGREDIENTS:

Chia Seeds	⅔ cup
Nut Milk	**2** cups
Cinnamon	
Raw, Organic Honey	

I bring this recipe to parties often. The coolness of this recipe is great as a dessert with hot soups. Also, the creamy texture supports ice cream cravings.

❄ SERVED COLD

🍓 SWEET

1   Mix all of the ingredients and chill for 3 hours. Drizzle with honey.

Conscious Cereal

(5 Minutes)

*Great crunchy
cereal substitute.*

❄ SERVED COLD

🍓 SWEET

INGREDIENTS:

**A Variety Of Your
Favorite Nuts & Seeds** | **1** cup

Almonds, Walnuts, Pecans, Brazil Nuts,
Macadamia Nuts, Pumpkin Seeds

Coconut Milk

Cinnamon

Raw Organic Honey

1 Crush the nuts and seeds to your liking.

2 Top with nut milk, cinnamon, and honey.

3 Enjoy!

Jicama, Citrus & Watercress Salad

(10 Minutes)

INGREDIENTS:

Pomegranate Juice	¼ cup
Seasoned Rice Vinegar	1 tbl
Agave Nectar	1½ tspn
Dijon Mustard	1½ tspn
Lime Zest, Finely Grated	½ tspn
Olive Oil	½ cup
Salt & Freshly Ground Pepper	
Red Grapefruit	1
Navel Oranges	2
Jicama Peeled And Cut Into 2-By-1/4-Inch Matchsticks	1 lb
Watercress Thick Stems Discarded	2 bunches
Pomegranate Seeds	⅓ cup

A fresh salad that gives you prebiotics to support digestion.

❄ SERVED COLD

🍓 SWEET

1 In a blender, combine the pomegranate juice, vinegar, agave nectar, mustard, and lime zest. With the machine on, add the oil in a thin stream and blend until emulsified. Season the dressing with salt and pepper.

2 Using a sharp knife, peel the grapefruit and oranges, removing all of the bitter white pith. Working over a bowl, cut in between the membranes to release the sections. Add the jicama, watercress, and pomegranate seeds to the bowl. Add the dressing, toss gently, and serve right away.

Reset Shake

(5 Minutes)

This shake can help you rebalance your liver with just one smoothie! I crave this shake when my body is needing more nutrients.

❄ SERVED COLD

🍓 SWEET

INGREDIENTS:

Apple	**1** half
Peeled Lime	**1**
Fresh Spinach	**1** cup
Hemp Seeds	**1** tbl
Coconut Water	**½** cup
Coconut Milk	**1** cup
Peeled Ginger	**1** inch
Fresh Mint	**¼** cup
Ice	

1 Blend and enjoy!

Shredded Carrot Salad

(5 Minutes)

INGREDIENTS:

Lemon Juice	1 tbl
Olive Oil, Extra-Virgin	1 tbl
Garlic, Minced, Small	½ clove
Sea Salt	⅛ tspn
Freshly Ground Pepper, To Taste	
Carrots, Shredded	1 cup
Fresh Dill, Chopped	1½ tbl
Scallion, Chopped	1 tbl

I crave this side dish. Broccoli and carrot shredded in a to-go bag for more convenience.

❄ SERVED COLD

🍓 SWEET

1 Whisk lemon juice, oil, garlic, sea salt, and pepper to taste in a medium bowl. Add carrots, dill, and scallion; toss to coat.

Yogurt with Almonds & Honey

(5 Minutes)

INGREDIENTS:

Vegan Yogurt, Plain	1 cup
Almonds, Crushed	¼ cup
Drizzle Of Raw, Organic Honey	

Great meal for breakfast on hot summer mornings.

❄ SERVED COLD

🍓 SWEET

1   Combine all ingredients and enjoy.

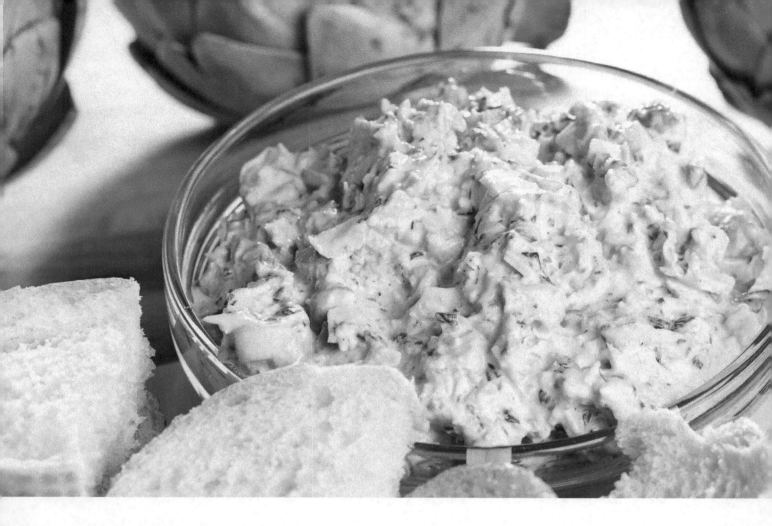

Snacks

Conscious Nutrition Snacks are recommended between meals only if you are hungry. Once you get your blood sugar balanced, snacks may be less needed.

Enjoy!

Artichoke Dip

(30 Minutes)

A great conscious snack to bring to a party, so you have something to eat.

🔥 SERVED HOT

🌙 SAVORY

INGREDIENTS:

(14-oz) Artichoke Hearts, Drained And Chopped	**1** can
(10-oz) Frozen Spinach, Chopped (Thawed And Drained)	**1** package
(8-oz) Plain Whole Fat Yogurt	**1**
Shredded Mozzarella Cheese	**1** cup
Green Onion, Chopped	**¼** cup
Garlic, Minced	**1** clove
Red Bell Peppers (Optional)	**2** tbl

1 Preheat oven to 350° F.

2 In a bowl, use emulsifying blender on all ingredients except bell peppers and mix well. Pour into a casserole dish.

3 Bake 20-25 minutes. Sprinkle with chopped bell peppers and serve with rice crackers or veggies.

Kale Chips

(15 Minutes)

INGREDIENTS:

Kale, Chopped	1	bunch
Lemon Juice	1	tbl
Olive Oil	2	tbl
Sea Salt	¼	tspn

*Amazing snack to satisfy
our crunch craving.*

⬡ SERVED HOT

◗ SAVORY

1   Preheat oven to 350° F. Line a non-insulated cookie sheet with parchment paper.

2   With a knife or kitchen shears, carefully remove the leaves from the thick stems and tear into bite size pieces. Wash and thoroughly dry kale with a salad spinner. Drizzle kale with oil and sprinkle with sea salt. For more flavors, try cayenne pepper or garlic powder.

3   Bake until the edges brown but are not burnt; 10-15 minutes.

Hummus

(10 Minutes)

*Try making your own
hummus vs. the store for less
artificial ingredients.*

❄ SERVED COLD

🌙 SAVORY

INGREDIENTS:

(16-oz) Chickpeas Or Garbanzo Beans	1 can
Liquid From Can Of Chickpeas	¼ cup
Lemon Juice (Depending On Taste)	3–5 tbl
Tahini	1½ tbl
Garlic, Crushed	2 cloves
Sea Salt	½ tspn
Olive Oil	2 tbl

1 Combine ingredients in emulsifying Blender and blend. Just remember to put in your thicker ingredients first, like the chickpeas and tahini.

2 Add in artichoke hearts, basil, cilantro, or red peppers for a variety of flavors.

Organic Guacamole

(10 Minutes)

INGREDIENTS:

ddd Ingredients:

Avocados, Ripe Organic	4
Vidalia Or Sweet Yellow Onion, Organic, Finely Chopped	1 medium
Roma Or Beefsteak Tomato, Organic	1 medium
Lime, Organic	1 large
Jalapeno Peppers, Organic Finely Chopped (Seeds Removed)	2 small
Garlic, Organic Finely Minced	2 cloves
Sea Salt, Organic (To Taste)	
Ground White Pepper, Organic (To Taste)	
Cilantro, Fresh Organic Finely Chopped (Stems Removed)	1 bunch

Scoop With Vegetables Such As; Cucumbers, Red Peppers, Hot Carrots, And Much More.

This snack is wonderful in the mid-afternoon with vegetables to keep your mind clear and energy up.

❄ SERVED COLD

🌙 SAVORY

1   Cut all 4 avocados into halves. Remove pits. With a sharp knife, score each half length and crosswise to form cubes. Scrape out each avocado half into a large mixing bowl.

2   Roll lime on counter top to allow juice to surface. Cut lime in half and squeeze juice over avocados — careful not to drop any seeds into your bowl.

3   Add onion, tomato, jalapeno, garlic, and cilantro into bowl. Mix vigorously with a wooden spoon or blend for extra creaminess. Add sea salt and pepper to taste. If you prefer a more whipped guacamole, try using a hand mixer to whip some of the avocados before adding all of the other ingredients.

4   Scoop with veggies and enjoy!

Ants on a Log

(3 Minutes)

*For the kid in
all of us*

❄ SERVED COLD

🍓 SWEET

INGREDIENTS:

Celery, Chopped	**1** bunch	
Cashew Butter	**4** tbl	
Raisins, Organic	**1–2** tbl	

Another Favorite Is Banana Boats:

1 Slice bananas in half and top with almond butter and honey.

Nut Butter (Make Your Own):

1 Add either almonds, cashews, walnuts, macadamia, or pecans (or combine a couple) in an emulsifying blender. Blend for a longer duration depending on what texture you prefer.

Banana Ice Cream

(5 Minutes)

A super supportive dessert to help with sugar cravings and sustain your energy.
This dessert is one of my favorites to serve for friends.

INGREDIENTS:

Bananas, Frozen	**4**
Cinnamon	1 dash
Nutmeg	1 dash
Vanilla	1 tspn
Ice	

❄ SERVED COLD

🍓 SWEET

1 BLEND and Enjoy!

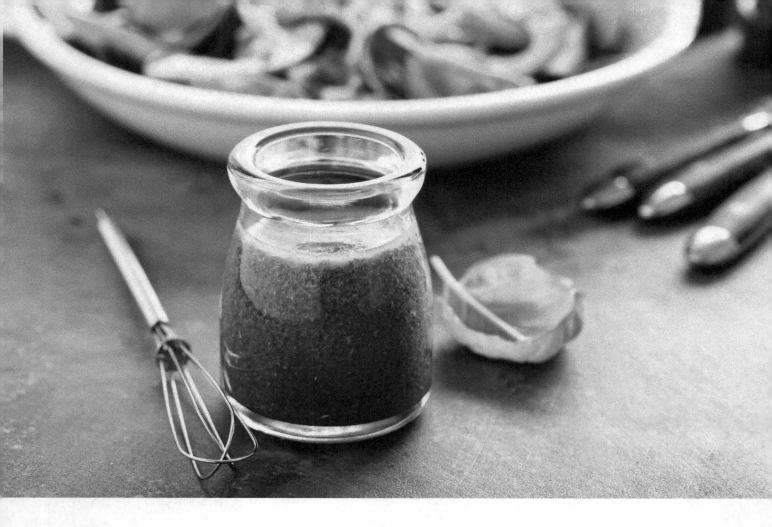

Dressings

Always have a bottle of already made dressing handy for you in predicaments. My favorite is Healthy Vinaigrette from the brand Braggs. And when your creativity strikes, try these recipes for a fresh alternative.

Enjoy!

Black Pepper Pesto Salad Dressing

(5 Minutes)

*Great dressing for
any salad.*

❄ SERVED COLD

🌙 SAVORY

PESTO

Garlic, Clove	1 large
Pine Nuts, Toasted	½ cup
Basil Leaves, Fresh, Packed	1 cup
Coarsely Ground Black Pepper	1½ tspn
Olive Oil, Virgin	¾ cup

VINAIGRETTE

Olive Oil, Extra Virgin	1 cup
Red Wine Vinegar	¼ cup
Black Pepper Pesto	¼ cup

1 Combine garlic, pine nuts, basil, and black pepper in an emulsifying blender and pulse a few times. Slowly add olive oil while continuing to pulse; should remain slightly course.

2 Can be tossed with pasta, served as a veggie dip, or create the vinaigrette and drizzle over steamed vegetables.

Mayonnaise

(5 Minutes)

INGREDIENTS:

Organic Free Range Egg	1
Garlic, Minced	½ tspn
Lemon Juice	1 tbl
Prepared Yellow Mustard	1 tspn
Olive Oil	¾ cup
Sea Salt & Pepper (To Taste)	

Store bought mayonnaise uses lower quality oils. Try making your own to add zest and creaminess with your meals.

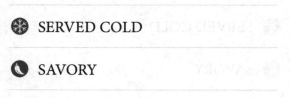

❄ SERVED COLD

🌙 SAVORY

1 Combine the organic free-range egg, garlic, lemon juice, and mustard in the container of an emulsifying blender. Blend until smooth, then blend on low speed while pouring oil into the blender in a fine stream as the mixture emulsifies and thickens.

Carrot/Ginger Dressing

(5 Minutes)

Drizzle this on a salad or any of your roasted veggies.

INGREDIENTS:

Carrot, Chopped	**1**
Ginger	**1** in
Rice Vinegar	**3** tbl
Sesame Oil	**3** tbl
Water	**1** tbl
Honey	**1** tbl
Bragg's Liquid Amino Acid	**1** tbl
Sea Salt	**1** tspn

❄ SERVED COLD

🍓 SWEET

1 Blend and enjoy!

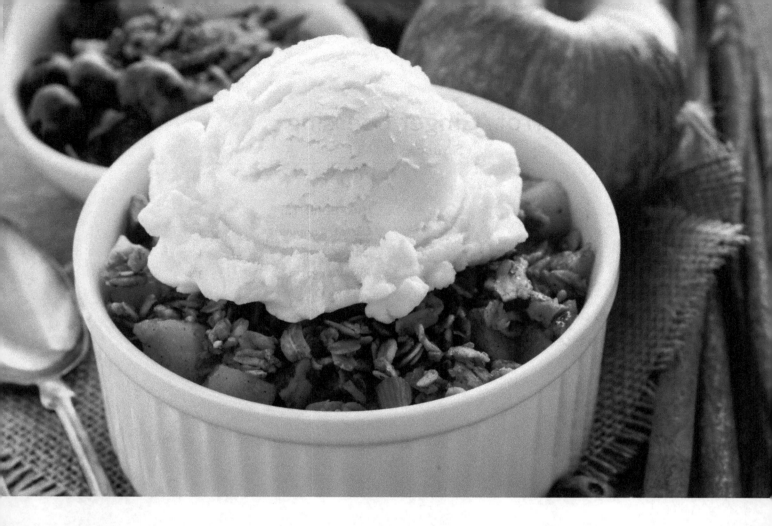

Desserts

Conscious Nutrition Desserts include whole and organic ingredients. Ask yourself if food is replacing another emotional need that is not being met?

Enjoy!

Almond Flour Madeleines

(20 Minutes)

*A wonderful dessert!
This dessert will make you feel like
you are in Europe!*

🔥 SERVED HOT

🍓 SWEET

INGREDIENTS:

Almond Flour	1½ cups
Organic Cane Sugar	½ cup
Brown Rice Flour	¼ cup
Arrowroot Powder	3 tbl
Baking Powder	2 tspn
Sea Salt	½ tspn
Coconut Oil (Plus Extra For Brushing)	½ cup
Hot Water	¼ cup
Pure Vanilla Extract	2 tspn
Ground Flaxseed	2 tbl
Water	5 tbl
Organic Powdered Sugar For Dusting	

1 Preheat oven to 325 degrees Fahrenheit. Brush 2-3 madeleine trays with coconut oil. In a large bowl, add almond flour, cane sugar, rice flour, arrowroot, baking powder, and sea salt. Whisk until no clumps remain.

2 In a separate bowl, whisk together coconut oil and vanilla extract. Set aside. In a small bowl, whisk together the flaxseed and 5 tablespoons water to form an "egg". Let set for 5 minutes. Add flax egg to the bowl of coconut oil and vanilla and whisk together. Once mixed well, add to the dry ingredients and mix with a rubber spatula until smooth. Slowly pour in hot water, stirring as you go. Once completely smooth, add approximately ½ tablespoon batter to each madeleine mold.

3 Bake for 14-16 minutes, until golden brown along edges. Rotate tray halfway through. Once cooled, remove cookies from pan, loosening with a butter knife along edges if needed. Transfer to a plate. Add powdered sugar to a sifter or sieve and sprinkle each cookie with the powdered sugar. Serve immediately or store in a jar for 1 week on the counter.

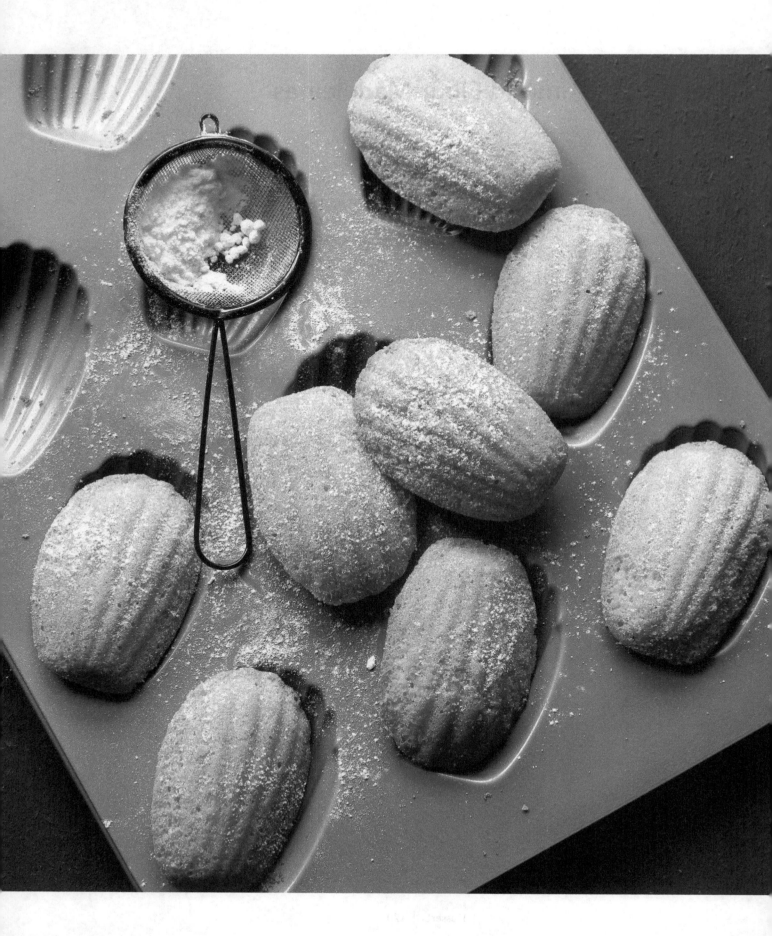

My Grandma's Apple Crisp (Healthy Version)

(40 Minutes)

My dear Grandma Kloppel wore a purple wig and played poker. This was her signature dish (with extra butter), this was her ticket into any party.

🔥 SERVED HOT

🍓 SWEET

INGREDIENTS:

Chopped Apples, Any Variety	**1** lb
Cinnamon	**2** tbl
Almond Milk	**1** cup
Oatmeal	**½** cup

1 4 apples (firm variety is better baking with) cut and spread into glass pan. Top with cinnamon and crushed nuts (almonds, pecans, and walnuts). Use emulsifying blender to crush. Pour 10-oz of coconut milk over.

2 Add love for your Grandma.

3 Bake at 425° F for 30 minutes.

Pumpkin Puree

(60 Minutes)

Supports healthy digestion when you may be experiencing loose stool or chronic digestive issues.

INGREDIENTS:

Pie pumpkins
(sugar, cheese, jack-be-little)

❄ SERVED COLD

🍓 SWEET

1 Wash and dry the outside of the pumpkins. Cut off the stems; then, cut the pumpkins in half from top to bottom. Scoop out all the seeds and strings. Cut the pumpkin pieces in half once more to create quarters. Place the pieces on a baking sheet, face down and bake at 350° F for 45-60 minutes. Allow the pumpkins to cool 10 minutes. Then, scoop out the cooked pulp and discard the skins.

2 Add into an emulsifying blender until smooth. Put the puree in a cheesecloth-lined colander over a bowl, and refrigerate overnight. (This will allow excess water to drain from the pumpkin so the puree isn't overly watery).

3 Use your pumpkin puree right away, store it in the refrigerator for use within the next week, or freeze it for use within the next year.

Stir it into oatmeal, make a creamy dessert, stir it into applesauce, use it in soups and chilies, or as a delicious ravioli filling.

Raw Chocolate Cake

(15 Minutes)

*Very decadent and full
of healthy fat.*

❄ SERVED COLD

🍓 SWEET

INGREDIENTS:

Walnuts, Raw, Unsoaked	1½ cups
Sea Salt	1 dash
Medjool Dates, Pitted, Unsoaked	12
Unsweetened Cocoa Or Carob Powder	⅓ cup
Vanilla Extract	½ tspn
Avocado, Smashed	¾ cup
Water	2 tspn
Fresh Raspberries For Garnish (Optional)	½ cup

1 Blend walnuts and sea salt in emulsifying blender until finely ground. Add dates, avocado, cocoa powder, and vanilla; process until mixture begins to stick together. Add the water and process briefly.

2 Transfer to a serving plate and form into a 5-inch round cake. Chill for 2 hours.

3 Decorate the cake and plate with fresh raspberries before serving, if desired.

4 Covered with plastic wrap, cake will keep refrigerated for 3 days or two weeks in the freezer.

Raw Chocolate Pudding

(10 Minutes)

INGREDIENTS:

Water	¼ cup
Honey, Local, Raw, Organic, (An Alternative Would Be Vanilla Stevia Instead Of Agave, Add To Suit Your Taste)	¼ cup
Cacao Powder, Raw, Organic (Purchase Raw Cacao Powder, Don't Use Coco Powder Or Anything Cooked)	½ cup
Avocados, Ripe	**2** medium/large

When you need chocolate and creamy all in one.

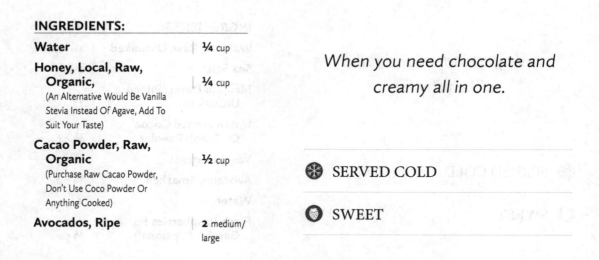

SERVED COLD

SWEET

1   Use the emulsifying blender to blend the first three items a bit first, then while blending, add pieces of avocado and fold in as necessary. It gets rather sticky, but with patience, it will turn into a nice pudding consistency. It only takes a few minutes and you can chill in the refrigerator.

Other Choices:

1   Though it's perfect just as it is, here are some options you can consider:
Use a fruit garnish
Use vanilla stevia instead of agave
Leave some chunks of avocado for texture and interest
Could add cacao nibs for crunch
Could add coconut
Could add almond butter

Rice Pudding

(8 Minutes)

This is one of my favorite desserts or breakfast idea.

🔥 SERVED HOT

🍓 SWEET

INGREDIENTS:

Leftover Cooked Rice (Preferably Basmati Or Jasmine)	¾ cup
Vanilla Almond Milk	¾ cup
Ground Cinnamon	¼ tspn
Almond Or Vanilla Extract	¼ tspn
Sliced Almonds, Roasted	¼ cup
Diced Apples Or Pears	¼ cup

1 Combine rice, almond milk, cinnamon and extract in a small saucepan. Turn heat to medium and bring to a simmer, stirring occasionally.

2 Reduce heat to medium-low and simmer gently for 4 to 5 minutes, until milk is thicker and rice is a bit creamy.

3 To serve, place in a bowl, top with sliced almonds and diced fruit.

Strawberry-Rhubarb Crisp

(50 Minutes)

INGREDIENTS:

Gluten-Free Rolled Oats	1 cup
Almond Flour	½ cup
Pure Maple Syrup	¼ cup
Coconut Oil	¼ cup
Ground Cinnamon	¼ tspn
Himalayan Salt Or Sea Salt	¼ tspn
Rhubarb Fresh Or Thawed	1½ cup
Strawberries	1 cup
Coconut Sugar	⅓ cup

*DESSERT! or
even a great breakfast for an
oatmeal substitute.
This crisp satisfies all of your
taste buds and cravings from the
Conscious Nutrition Cravings
Book, such as hot, sweet
and creamy.*

🔥 SERVED HOT

🍓 SWEET

1 Preheat the oven to 375 degrees Fahrenheit and lightly oil an 8x8 baking dish.

2 In a large bowl, mix together oats, almond flour, coconut sugar, cinnamon, and salt.

3 Stems the leaves off of the rhubarb, being sure to trim at least ¼ inch off the ends of rhubarb. Chop the rhubarb into ½-1 inch pieces, placing into a medium bowl. Slice the strawberries and add to the bowl. Add maple syrup and coconut oil and mix well.

4 If using frozen rhubarb, you will need to transfer the mixture to a pot and heat over medium heat as the coconut oil will solidify against the cold rhubarb. Heat until melted and remove from heat.

5 Add the fruit mixture to the dry ingredients and stir until well combined. Transfer to the baking dish.

6 Bake for 30 -45 minutes or until the topping has crisped and turned golden brown.

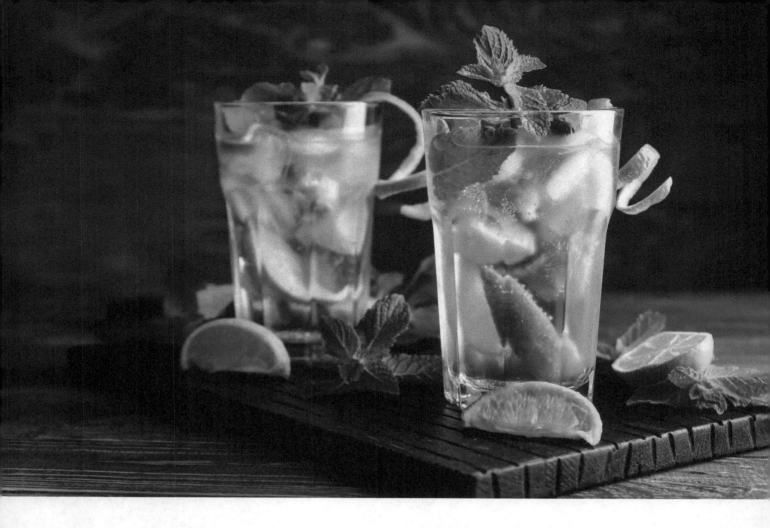

Drinks

To help quench your thirst without the added artificial ingredients.

Enjoy!

Mojito

(5 Minutes)

Refreshing and hydrating drink.

❄ SERVED COLD

🍋 SOUR

INGREDIENTS:

Club Soda	**4** oz
Mint Leaves, Fresh	**4-8**
Honey	**1** tspn
Lime Juice	**2** tspn
Splash Of Water & Ice	

1 Muddle the mint, add in honey, lime juice, ice, and soda. Enjoy!

Root Beer

(5 Minutes)

INGREDIENTS:

Club Soda	**8** oz
Root Beer Liquid Extract (To Taste)	
Cinnamon	
Organic Apple Cider Vinegar	**2** oz

My favorite 'soda' and this recipe is a great alternative

❄ SERVED COLD

🍋 SOUR

1   Add ice cubes to your glass with 8-oz of either club soda or Kombucha.

2   Splash 2-oz of organic apple cider vinegar into the glass.

3   Add root beer extract to taste.

Spring Soda

(5 Minutes)

Something refreshing for you to have versus just water.

INGREDIENTS:

Mint Leaves, Fresh	¼ cup
Cucumber, Slices	4-5
Club Soda, Plain Or Lime	
Lime Wedge	

❄ SERVED COLD

🍋 SOUR

1. Place mint at the bottom of a Collins glass and top with ice.

2. Line the sides of the glass with cucumber slices.

3. Top with soda, ice, and lime wedges.

Dandy Hot Toddy

(7 Minutes)

A wonderful night cap. This night cap is great to help with sugar cravings and support heart health.

INGREDIENTS:

Dandy Blend Or 2 Bags Of Dandelion Tea	**2** tbl
Coconut Cream	**2** tbl
Honey, Raw, Organic	**½** tspn
Cinnamon	**1** dash

🔥 SERVED HOT

🍓 SWEET

1 Brew tea or add hot water to the Dandy blend.

2 Add coconut cream and honey.

3 Sprinkle with cinnamon.

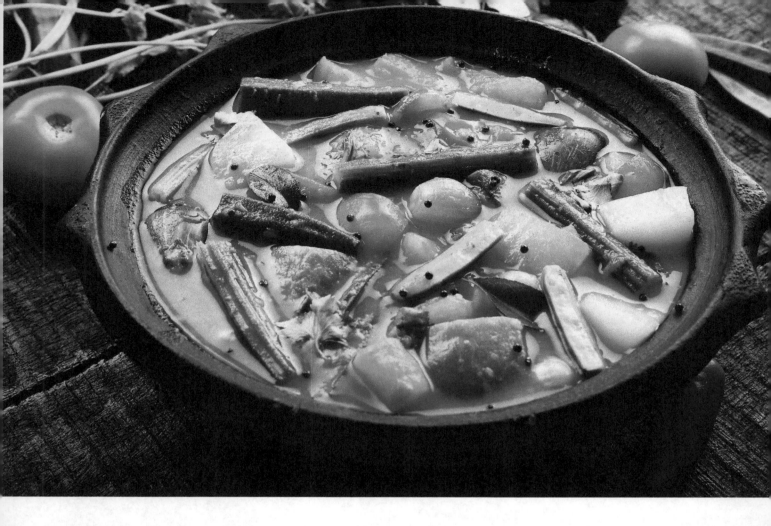

Appendix

Here you can find an index of recipes listed by name and a place to add future recipes from Conscious Nutritions.

Contents

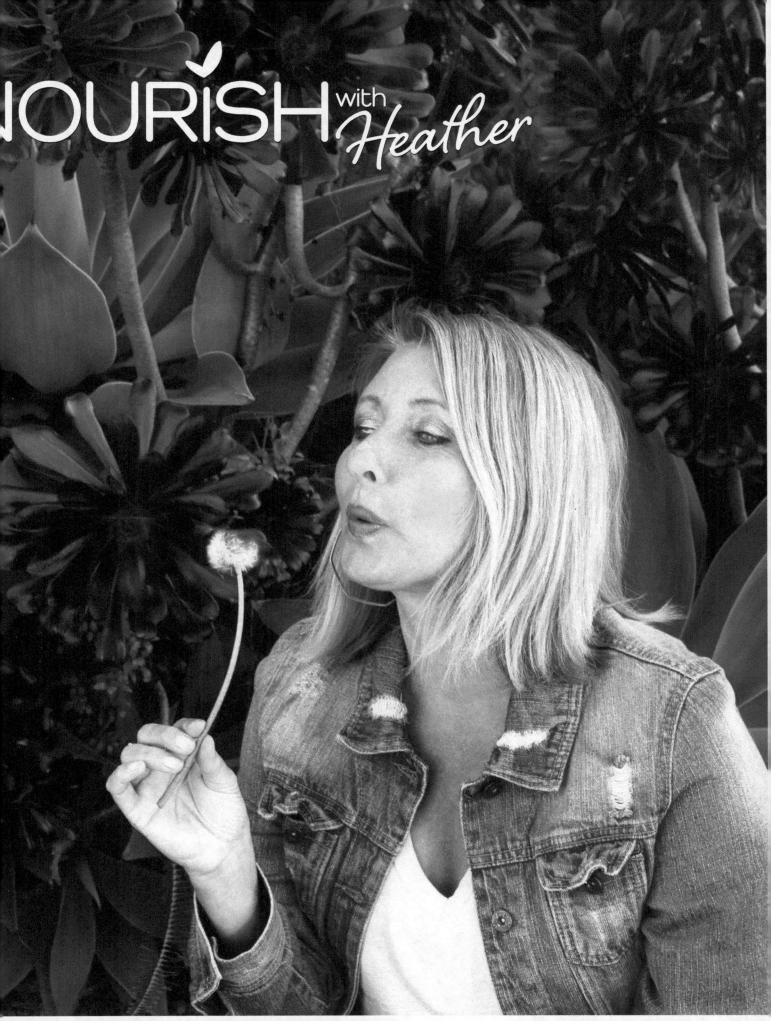

CPSIA information can be obtained
at www.ICGtesting.com
Printed in the USA
BVHW05022709032 2
630907BV00006B/36

9 780578 351599